A PETIT MAL
A MOTHER'S HEALING
LOVE SONG
ANA MARÍA CABALLERO

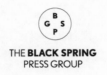

THE **BLACK SPRING**
PRESS GROUP

(BUT IN THE LAMPLIGHT,
DOWNED WITH LIGHT BROWN HAIR!)

'THE LOVE SONG OF J. ALFRED PRUFROCK',
T.S. ELIOT

First published in 2023
An Eyewear Publishing book, The Black Spring Press Group
Maida Vale, London w9
United Kingdom

Typesetting User Design, Illustration and Typesetting, UK
Photo credit Adrian Avila

The author has requested the publisher use American
spelling and grammar wherever possible in this edition

ISBN-13 978-1-915406-08-8

A PETIT MAL

CONTENTS

JUDGE'S CITATION

To begin, in naming a winner for the Beverly Prize, I have to say how struck I was by the sheer variety and daring of the manuscripts. I was asked to choose "the best" from a stunning list of very different works—from poetry to novels to essays to memoir to short stories. How to compare? How to choose?

I looked for manuscripts that stayed with me after an initial read-through. Voices that slyly demanded attention stylistically as well as thematically. I looked for stories which surprised me, but which also cried out for a larger public. Many congratulations are due to these shortlisted writers, because each one absolutely fulfills these criteria. Thank you for giving me such stimulating reading over these past months!

My winning choice is Ana Maria Caballero's extraordinary work of creative non-fiction, *A Petit Mal*.

This is a precisely-calibrated work of non-fiction. Caballero writes about her quest to understand her son's epilepsy. *A Petit Mal* is a difficult book, asking questions that do not have clear answers. The author weaves poetry, stark statement, and stream-of-consciousness into a narrative voice of rare empathy and honesty.

Whose story is this, Caballero asks, because she is telling her own story, but also, inevitably, her son's. As a family, she and her husband seek alternative healing possibilities for their suffering child—a journey which takes them to a wide array of "witch doctors", as she comes to call the team of doctors, healers, and even the convincingly helpful veterinarian. But of course, by writing the exact details of her days, by discussing her son's various treatments, she also inevitably involves other people and their stories. How can one writer make sense of memory and experience at all? Is a literary form useful for such exploration? How can we remain honest, while interpreting the way other people choose to live?

We feel Caballero's confusion, her desperation, when she writes, "*What to believe, we ask. All of it: for now, believe all the doctors say. It must be coming, nearing, we say, the pierce of sharp lamplight.*" Note the lack of question marks in that section. In fighting for answers, Caballero experiments with the very idea of questions. She adjusts punctuation, plays with space on the page, makes asides with witty footnotes, in a constant and successful challenge to smoothly straight-forward memoir. Nothing about her son's journey was smooth, and as a creative work, Caballero clearly lays out the manuscript as one large query—about the medical establishment, about individual life, about healing and spirituality.

In focusing on her son's story, Caballero brings in not only her own fears and interests, but also those of her family, her friends, and those of writers she admires. This extended literary family forms a skeletal support for the book. Caballero spirals repeatedly back to T.S. Eliot's poem 'The Love Song of J.Alfred Prufrock.' Circling the core story of her son's struggle, Caballero weaves strands of these extended stories from personal to literary and back again.

Caballero is writing her way through the experience as a poet, creating a deep, spiritually complex, self-questioning work of non-fiction. She writes: "I will not miss/seizure of boy when/gone But I will miss/writing of book when/done." As I miss reading this book, now that I am done. It circles, dares, and intrigues the reader, and for these qualities *A Petit Mal* is the winning manuscript for the Beverly Prize.

Lisa Pasold

For Lolo, who is grand,
and for Elizabeth, whom I miss.

Note to the reader

vs., &, x/y, ( )

These textual markings are used as separators between sections throughout the text, each serving the same function but connecting in symbolic ways with the events taking place in their respective chapters.

daimon diamond monad I
Adam Kadmon in the sky

Ronald Johnson

1

The medical clinical procedure by which an illness is diagnosed will not be presented here. Not really. Really: the disruptive experience of it. Not personal illness but illness of other, illness of child. Do not stop reading for fear this will be sad. It will not. Not the entire way through. No longer than the duration of moment, of event. Sad because of child, and even not being parent, sadness wrought by ill child is experienced vividly, is readily accessible, in adult form. Even when not experienced directly as a specific sequence of events within own singular story of life. Even when read.

Eventually, I will make you happy. But it will be a process. A procedure, but not a medical clinical one, not even, entirely, a holistic one, because "holistic" can mean "complete" and procedure here will not be complete. Here, "procedure" will mean "progression," as in on-going and beyond the confines of material book.

"Holistic" may also mean "whole," as in "sound." Process will not be sound in the way completion is sound, is circular, is whole. Gradually, increasingly, we will name procedure together, procedure I will present here for you. We will get there. Please read. Whatever it is, we will name it together. The process of sad to happy to sad to happy is so important. Because nothing need change outside. The coffee, so long as already good, can continue to be same good coffee. Here, drink, warm coffee waiting warmly in my hands.

The event, though. The event is important. The event that marks an external change, a change that extends inside, within the bounds of material skin. The event, the fulcrum about which the story pivots, the moment that launches this specific sequence of story of life.

I am able to name a single event. I am. The single event of playing soccer with boy and all of a sudden ball is mine without slide-tackling boy, and I hear from behind boy say, *it's happening*. Boy clutches net, net moves with him, and he moves from side to side with net, net that moves with him. I hold boy by waist even though swaying is slight and look at boy while I kneel on ground so that I can see with entire eyes entire face of boy at same height and boy is laughing hard, wild, when he says, *it stopped*. Boy runs to take ball from me because boy is fine. Back to fine. Return to fine. Return—from where.

The event, the moment, the experience: occurrence fused with apprehension of fear. Fear because intuition. Intuition of mother, of human mother, but also animal, animal parent. Something is wrong. The event, pinned: the incident. But, the what within, the how within, the why—not known.

The event, the moment, the instant of decision of hospital. Of packing to go and awareness of stay. Of the coming days inside hospital. Days to come, preemptively perceived—

The madwoman in the house. Socks, underwear, chargers. Books, I pack two. Two new books because I knew. Now, when I write, I can remember how painstakingly I knew. Of the days to come, I knew.

But also, less exact: the urgency of hospital was not warped by fear of immediate risk to life. Rather: a faint detection of unnamed condition entering boy's life, to our family's life. Because of this detection, I had a timid awareness that we would all, eventually, survive, I was able to play music in car, able to drive.

Timid awareness, remote from the active knowledge of active unknowing. Slight, voiceless awareness, a sigh behind the structure of words. Faint awareness, thought unformed, that yet still informs, guides, helps maneuver the material movement of muscle, of bone, of being, who, within skin, was able to function and go.

vs.

In ER, we are seen by French doctor, which is unusual and relevant because doctor asks boy if he likes any French soccer teams. Boy is wearing Italian soccer jersey.

Yes, Paris Saint-Germain, boy says.

Ah, doctor says, *you like* PSG. *And you also like Juventus, ah*.

Boy is wearing soccer jersey with the number and name of Juan Guillermo Cuadrado, a well-known Colombian striker who plays for Juventus, a team from Italian city of Turin.

Yes.

French doctor asks, *is Cuadrado still alive*.

The French doctor is making a dark joke: *is Cuadrado still alive*. This question is a joke. A question asked because a Colombian soccer player was murdered nearly thirty years ago as gruesome, ghastly punishment for scoring a self-goal in a world cup. The 1994 Italian World Cup. My husband, boy, I are Colombian. A fact we had already shared with doctor.

All this important because boy laughs, but the joke, the question, is not funny. The doctor's joke is not funny. Not even bad funny. Perhaps uncomfortable funny, perhaps uncanny inappropriate funny, perhaps adult offensive funny. But not kid funny, and boy laughs, boy who does not, I am certain, recognize joke. Boy laughs a lot.

My voice: *it's happening.*

And he, emergency room pediatric doctor who recognizes he should not have said what he just said knows, too, that "it" is happening. Doctor orders CT Scan.

VS.

The power by which CT Scan is ordered. The years of school. The decades. Position earned via disproportionate time on foot. Other children in other ER rooms. Other bad jokes. Other silences. Other bursts of laughter.

Give this child scan, this, not that. Boy laughs loud: laughs a laugh that is off. Silence does not equal scan.

VS.

The CT Scan is clear. No, not clear. It is "unremarkable." Medically, clinically, unremarkable is what bedside prayers are made of. Unremarkable boy under the unquiet, disquiet whir of CT Scan. What's more, the report goes—

"The globes and orbits appear within normal limits."

Normal globes, normal orbits, normal limits within boundaries of boy. An incidental finding: scan reveals empty *sella turcica.* The doctors try to explain.[1] An extra molar. A difference in eye color. Discolored nipples. No, they don't mention nipples. I mention it to myself inside my head to try to comprehend "incidental" in terms of body. My high-school best-friend's incidentally humungous nipples. Incidental is not what bedside prayers are made of. It is vague. Why mention it. Incidentally

---

1   They are bad at explaining, I find.

your boy, your boy in ER, has empty *sella* in brain. Should the *sella* be half-empty, doctor. Or, rather, half-full.

I go online. Doctors insist, do not go online. Online, I learn. Reputable websites belonging to reputable hospitals. I avoid forums, incidentally, at all cost. An empty *sella* refers to a cavity, the *sella turcica,* that is actually full of cerebrospinal fluid in base of skull. In Latin, *sella turcica* means *Turkish seat*. The *sella* a seat for the pituitary gland, headquarters of hormone production. Online it says that this is what doctors think, what doctors consider, imagine, believe.

An online search for *Turkish seat* yields billions of images of ultra-low rectangular loveseats covered in mostly red fabrics. Another billion images of seats in Turkish Airlines. Nothing summons cavity.

Who names the lesser parts of body. A Turkish seat buried within brain of boy. Visible by lamplight of CT Scan. Incidental, but not unremarkably so.

vs.

We are admitted.

vs.

Two new books inside the parked car.

vs.

I am familiar with hospital because of recently. A friend who is a recent friend has a baby, baby Anaya, recently diagnosed with cancer. With stage four neuroblastoma. Baby is eighteen months when diagnosed. Cancer is in brain, in abdomen, in marrow of her bones. Anaya whose name resembles mine.

Whose name also recalls place in paternal grandparent's native land of Lebanon. Place where grandparents are, incidentally, when diagnosis is received by them via call.

My friend terms hospital *The Terminal* because being there is like being at airport, eternally, with baby. Entertaining while waiting for something other to happen, to arrive, to land upon. For example: insertion of substance. For example: analysis of change of rate of heart, composition of blood, increase of temperature, result of exam delivered by physician on call, person with decades of school, proven to be good at withstanding hours of thinking while standing up.

There is really good coffee on ground floor. A café that makes Starbucks lattes. There, beyond unnamed reality of medical, clinical truth, lives the day-to-day. The unremarkable day-to-day. Different from truth of what may come, of what may land upon, of what's to arrive, but has not yet come. Good coffee a stated fact, substance inserted, absolute: Grande Latte in your hand. Truth that requires no physical scan.

vs.

One day before soccer-net-clutching-laughing-boy-hospital-dash-out-front-door, I take boy to pediatrician.

I say, *boy says he feels, sometimes, like he is going to fall. Boy laughs, leans back. But boy does not fall. I noticed it yesterday, two times yesterday, for the first time. Can we test boy's blood.*

Ok, pediatrician says. *Anything else.*

No. No fever, no boogers, no pain in any place. Eating, pooping, sleeping fine. Only the episodes. The feeling boy has that he will fall.

I'll check ear.

Ear. Pulse. Pressure. Bloodwork. All fine.

Vertigo, I say.

Maybe. But usually vertigo comes with near or actual fall.

Shall I go to hospital. Insist on scan.

No, wait.

Ok.

Fridays are bad at ER. *If it happens again, then go. You must insist on scan.*

Why.

They don't like to give kids scans.

Ok.

On car ride home, pediatrician calls.

You know, she says. *Maybe it is vertigo. Go to pharmacy, get boy a dose of Dramamine.*

Dramamine, I say.

Yes, Dramamine. Let's rule this out.

vs.

The hospital coffee shop that somehow is and is not Starbucks is closed on Sunday, which is my first morning waking up in hospital. So, I am sent to other coffee vendor in hospital that is open but has bad coffee.

Boy, of course, still upstairs. Still asleep. Still hooked up by twenty-four very thin color cables to EEG.

vs.

Incidentally, "epilepsy" is not a friendly word.

vs.

I'm not sad because boy is getting EEG. I'm grateful he's is granted EEG. The bed/couch that serves as bed for accompanying parent in hospital was/is fine. I read a lot of pages from one of my books. This book is pretty good, maybe even unmodifier/unmodified good. But the coffee is bad, and I am not awake. Not like I know from intuition of parent, of animal parent, that I want to be, ought to be, awake. This annoys me.

I am annoyed when husband calls and asks about boy. I say boy is fine. I ask husband to come quick and bring good coffee quick. I do not speak nicely. This makes husband think boy is not fine. I see myself not rising to the occasion. But seeing the not rising does not make me rise. I cannot rise because I am not awake. Because I am bad like bad coffee.

Boy is fine, I say. *Please come soon. Please bring good coffee.*

Words spoken on first morning at hospital. It makes no sense. I am impatient. I am annoyed. I do not feel sad. I am annoyed. Annoyance of husband, a man who answers to proper combined nouns of Nelson David.

I do not wish to be disturbed. I hold on to day-to-day.

vs.

Because EEG is clear, we need MRI. Of the brain and of the spine. Boy will need general anesthesia to lie supine.

vs.

To be clear, EEG is clear-clear. As in not incidental empty fuck shit fuck Turkish seat *sella* medical fuckface about-face unremarkable finding.

Did episodes happen while on EEG.

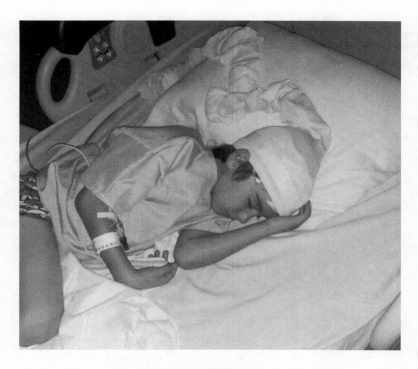

Yes, doctor, three. My boy pressed the red trigger episode button three times, one trigger for each of the times—

Each to each.

vs.

Boy has eight episodes, eight happenings, eight laughing wavering moments of imbalance on each of Saturday and of Sunday. On Monday morning we wake, and it is time for MRI. The nurse wakes me first. I ask the time. I ask if the coffee shop that is sort of Starbucks is open. She says yes. I ask if we can wait until I get one to wake my son and take him to MRI. She says yes.

She responds. When I come back with good coffee she asks, *ready*.

Ready, I say. A series with eight episodes.

Walls in MRI room painted bright, an underwater perky fish scene. Look at cool walls, I tell boy. Boy agrees they are cool. They are bright.

The MRI doctor is so very silly. He asks boy about what boy likes.

Messi, boy says.

Messi, or is it soccer that you like, doctor asks.

Insertion of substance. Boy with conclusively, instantaneously closed eyes. More good coffee left to drink held by my hand. Grandes are grand. Sequence of livable steps. It is fine to get an MRI.

vs.

The night before MRI, Sunday, I read about epilepsy on The Epilepsy Foundation's website. It is hard to read, as in academically difficult, but interesting. Focal seizures originate in one specific part of the brain. Generalized seizures mean entire electrical cerebral organ is off. Unknown next to seizures means of origin, of location unknown. As in indefinite source of electric impulse within perimeter of brain. The why for most seizures, the reason beneath, behind, generally, widely, occult.

Sometimes seizures make the person unaware of the seizure. Other times seizures make the person lose motor skills. Absence seizures are when the person leaves then comes back, as in leaves the actual world with mind but not body and is not aware of the leaving and then the coming back. Like a movie on pause. It does not know it is on pause.

Tonic-clonics are when the person convulses, on the floor, stiffens, turns blue, like in a horror film in which a victim is possessed. In the past, tonic-clonic seizures were called "grand mal seizures" and focal seizures were called "petit mal seizures." As in bad, but only a little.

Tonic-clonic and focal seizures were renamed in 2017 by a real-world organization named International League Against Epilepsy. A name that brings comic book hero conglomerations to mind.

Reading about seizures is interesting. New words, new uses of old words. "Onset" is brilliant in its simplicity, in its punch. A thought that originates within my right frontal lobe, where neurons finesse into words the emotional reactions elicited by life.

vs.

The night before MRI, Sunday night, I write a poem about Mother's Day. I am lying down next to boy in narrow, wheeled hospital bed and poem comes, and I know it is an old poem that has just arrived. And that it will not come again. And that there is some humor in it coming now. I keep saying humor.

There is some humor in it landing upon me now. This poetic lament of Mother's Day spoils. Perhaps there is humor because there is pathos. "Pathos" as in "bleak," but also "pathetic," *pathètique*. My laughter, like sudden seizure or sudden poem, comes abrupt, or not at all.

The poem belongs to a book I am writing called *Mammal*. All its poems numbered like this—

Mammal Thirty-One

I remind the one
Who is my husband
To bring a small gift soon
It will be the Day of the Mother
Role of Father Man
Husband Male
To procure
Box
Offering
For me to open
I tell him I am pliable
I point to trivial things
Explain how to go
He says he thought
Of something better
But he does not
Did not
Go
Am I sad
Am I literally sad
Am I sad poem sad
Am I proven right sad
Am I things will never change sad
Am I validator of bipartisan role of Mother
Sad
Mother's Day w/o box
W/o compensation
W/o plastic balloon
W/o breakfast on tray
W/o single drugstore rose unthorned
W/o picture to prove
To post to prove

Do I care
Do I want to care
Do I make myself care
Can I make it stop
Can I forgo
And if not
Can I go out
Can I buy a box
Bag my own goddam
Reward

vs.

The night before MRI, Sunday night, I finish reading the first of the two books I brought, Lily Hoang's *A Bestiary*. She writes about her day-to-day, also about things she learned from watching TV in the real world of her life.

Hoang also writes about jade bangles, the tighter a bangle is around wrist, the more valuable the wrist. The woman attached to wrist. About ways to get a small jade bangle onto wrist. Soap, oil, pain, will. The small green bangle, remarkable because of the fist's tacit contortion, remarkable in its ability to make the hand seem gentler, softer. I know the implications, the politics are all wrong, but also, I immediately know I will one day be on Canal Street pursuing impossible cold green jade for my improbably large hands. Not to punish my handspan but because onset of bangle so clear-cut in its sacrifice.

It feels good to finish book in real world. To read book and to finish. To comprehend book. To recognize life may always be good, because of book. To close book like an answer to which the question is book.

vs.

The night before MRI, Sunday night, my husband, Nelson David, calls. He is not well. He wants to talk. There is an underlying question, an undercurrent of want. It is my turn to be well. Don't ask those questions, I say. They are not good questions. It cannot be us, cannot be our fault. We must wait for MRI, then we will know. But let's think of this as condition, a condition we make part of life, of our good life.

I am the opposite of annoyed. Drawn toward, drawn by.

vs.

Two weeks before hospital. Before madwoman dash to hospital with boy who says he feels he may fall.

Two weeks before hospital, I travel to New Jersey to visit friend who gave hospital *The Terminal* name. Friend and her baby Anaya. In New Jersey for radiation treatment.

New Jersey is not that bad.

What is bad about New Jersey is the lack of suitable density. All the highways make things far. Make things same. And when you get to where you are going there's a big place to park, an ugly walk to walk. And where you are looks the same as from whence you came. So, you wonder if you were anywhere, went anywhere, are anywhere. Can possibly go anywhere, ever, at all. This process, abstracted from immediate reality of place, makes place interesting. Interesting thoughts of mind make place interesting as a temporary location of life.

I am glad to visit New Jersey. New Jersey is not that bad.

I am glad to see my friend in New Jersey, and I am glad to confirm she is in place that is not too bad. Anaya is doing so well. She is always happy, always, every day, naps, eats, plays. Friend and I have very good coffee. Marvel at the packed aisles, at the

rows, at the corridors of Whole Foods. Buy nothing but coffee.
Sit and eat nothing but coffee. Find good wine by the glass in
a place by Rutgers. Go for walk in freezing, handsomely land-
scaped park.

In New Jersey I begin to know something bad is coming
my way.

I have no proof of this knowing: having not said anything
to anyone, written anything down. It is, I realize, a moderate
knowing, a tug, temperate and kind. It is: dim lamplight. I will
explain further on why I was able to know. And what.

When she leaves New Jersey, I ask friend if she is relieved.

No, not at all. Actually, kind of miss it, she says. *Perhaps I have
Stockholm Syndrome.*

Perhaps all locations so long as temporary, as momentary,
as boundary, become similar to soothe, similar to hope, explicit
events that can be underlined, encircled, as good.

vs.

The underlying cause of fifty percent of seizures remains
unknown. This I learn from neurologist, whom I begin to
internalize as White Doctor because of white bald head atop
white small face atop white bald coat.

Unknown is presented as resolution, as a factual form of
knowing. It is clear fact, the clear fact is we do not know. This
fact, the patient may take home.

The medical, clinical word for "unknown" is not "remarkable." "Remarkable" is not a medical nor a clinical term. Only
"unremarkable" applies, is applicable, to organs of body of
person that are unremarkable because they work. The word for
conditions that find resolution in the inexplicable is "idiopathic."

Here are the terms above used in real world sentence of common words: my boy has unremarkable body organs, vital signs, blood that flows, yet lives, apparently, with a condition that is idiopathic.

Idio vs. pathic.

vs.

I call my life-long, alternative doctors "witch doctors" but they are not. They are doctors, with diplomas and such, connected to god. To God. To light, energy, flow. Each malady addressed in three parts: mind, body, soul. Antibiotics, antidepressants when necessary. But what, why, how, who, never ignored. Always, at onset, explored.

Doctors with whom, incidentally, I've worked for years.

vs.

The MRI comes back clear. Wait. Not clear, clear. Not EEG clear.

New neurologist, neurologist who's on duty on Monday, super friendly bubbly bouncy neurologist who delivers information, says MRI has something—actually. Something she would never have called. But they called it. They. The technicians who operate levers of MRI machine. They named it, the object—

"MRI revealed right centrum semi-ovale along the posterior superior aspect of the right frontal lobe (cortical dysplasia vs. small area of gliosis vs. hypomyelination)."

Versus vs. or. Or vs. either. Either vs. nor.

The bubbly bouncy neurologist would have never called it vs. the written, printed record in my hand that does. Industrious idiopathy.

vs.

I write to my army of witch doctors from the ground floor good coffee place while I wait for boy to emerge from MRI. Elsa, Sergio, Elizabeth, Lucila, Nelly.

The MRI *will be fine,* they say, *but he will need help, he will need zinc, magnesium, B6, B12, belladonna, selenium,* CBD *but the good kind, the kind compact with* TCH. *Check his blood, every week, check chemical imbalances, para-thyroid, Epstein-Barr, herpes, iron, heavy metals. No wheat, no sugar, no dairy, nothing that lives in the sea. Look up "le petit mal."*

They are going to give him medication, my witch doctors say. *Wait on the medication. As soon as you can, bring boy to me.*

Tráemelo.

vs.

The day after we emerge from hospital, I arrange a two-hour conversation with Sergio, master of astrology, dharma vs. karma, which includes consequences of food put repeatedly into mouth. He tells us boy has a Hamer point in his brain. An area of darkness formed from traumas generated in utero or within the first two years post-birth.

Sergio knows my story well. Sergio knows what happened while boy was in utero and pre-birth and post.

La muerte de mami y papi. Mami y papi convertidos en mamá y en papá, he says.

The day my daddy goes into hospital to get 1.5 liters of plasma drained from the hematoma in his brain I tell daddy I am pregnant with boy. I say, *Papi voy a tener un niño. Te tiene que ir bien.*

Daddy does not emerge. Not even unclear. Not ever. How, what, why, incidental. Who is the answer to which question, the only question, is whom.

vs.

I take five pregnancy tests the night I consider I may be heavy with child. All confirm I am incidentally unempty. The diagnosis is clear.

vs.

Before hospital discharge, we are told we must watch video on handling seizures at home. Roll patient to side. Check for loose items in mouth. Attempt removal of objects if found. Insert diazepam up rectum if seizure becomes cluster. "Cluster" in terms of seizure, like in the real world, means "collection," means "gathering," a clutter of motion, accruing, amassing. As in "horde," or "stampede."

Diazepam goes up the butt because throat passage may be shut. Injection uncertain during thrashing cluster attack. Boy may move fierce, even gripped by our hands.

vs.

Boy is six. Seven years ago, my daddy's mind left, gone.

Time as adult spans back, as it, as time, in present holds still. Grasps firm: bridges back. Wingspan of bird, bent out, back, then in, again out. Practical lever of physical, transfiguring flight, attached forever to one body, to core of singular bird.

Past attached to present, no matter how far past. Shapes and sways, despite seven years ago.

vs.

Emerge
is word,
    incidentally,
transformed.

vs.

Now, the speaking about. To family, to friends. The few.
To other doctors. The several. Many. Manifold.

I have been given an object: cortical dysplasia vs. small
area of gliosis vs. hypomyelination. An indeterminate object,
remarkable in its manifold forks of lexicon. To determine it,
it requires talk. I talk. I don't have object, determinate as one.

I have nothing, materially, so I talk.

vs.

*Give him the Keppra, and if the seizures go away, then we know they
were seizures*, says the foamy, fizzy neurologist after our right
frontal lobe gliosis vs. dysplasia vs. hypomyelination non-
diagnosis that foamy, fizzy neurologist would never have
called, but MRI report does call but does not call one thing.

A name vs. another name vs. another. Minute defect, abundant in words. Unclear, for boy, for us, this not-clear MRI.

The bubbly, the bouncy, the fizzy, the foamy, the super-
duper friendly neurologist is the second neurologist who visits
us in the hospital. I want her as doctor. Can I please have her
as doctor. No. Sorry. Our out-of-hospital neurologist must be
the first neurologist, White Doctor with white bald coat, white
bald terms. The one who sees us after clear, clear EEG, and says
it is time for MRI of the brain and of the spine. For which boy
must lie supine.

The first doctor, the White Doctor, our doctor, checks boy for birthmarks.

Birthmarks of skin, he says, *usually mean birthmarks of brain. The brain and the skin form simultaneously, in utero. Does your boy have marks.*

Yes, one on back thigh.

But doctor checks boy's back. Finds a mark I'd seen before but never gripped as mark. Was not awake aware of its presence. I feel embarrassed. The doctor and his entourage make note of the mark on back.

There is one on his thigh, I say, again.

The White Doctor looks, finds it, his medical crew smiles, takes note. Mom, mommy, was right. She knows her boy.

White Doctor gives boy a neurological physical, for which he employs little tools found in his little black doctor's bag. A rod shaped like giraffe with which to tap boy's knee with which to make knee snap. Knee snaps.

Physical is fine, doctor says.

Team writes.

Boy laughs.

I snap.

vs.

It's happening.

2

Elizabeth, Eli, the witch doctor at the heart of my former home of Bogotá, is bad at telephone. I know this, love her despite. At some off-set moment, she responds. Tells me: *le puse manitas*. I placed my hands on him. From far-off, Eli's figurative, far-flung hands are truthfully placed on boy.

There is something chemically off. Off-set. Not seizures, not birthmark of body, nor that of brain. Yet, electric. Foreign substance within boy's body, boy's body unable to properly, electrically process.

Tráemelo, she says, bring him to me.

vs.

Papi vs. papá. Mami vs. mamá. Birth vs. born. Borne vs. boy.

vs.

Boy will need a better story than that, Sergio says. Make one up. Make him the ending, he, boy, the happy ending in your better story. Tell it to him at night. In bed. Safe. Before sleep. The brain is open then, pliant as white cotton sheet.

Abuelo Fernando was not always in a wheelchair. Not always silent. He used to walk a lot, talk a lot, go places alone. He got sick because he fell on his head. He was old when he fell on his head. He fell on his head hard. His brain bled. The blood had nowhere to go. The doctors had to open a hole. Before they opened the hole, I told Abu Fernando I was pregnant with you. You were only five weeks old inside my belly. I told Abu Fernando that he had to do well in the hospital. That he had to come back okay after the doctors opened the hole.

The doctors opened his brain. Out came enough blood to fill a big bottle of soda. But Abu Fernando did not come out as himself. He is how you see him now. He spent a lot of time in the hospital. The doctors tried to understand what was wrong. But they could not. He was just too old. He had fallen on his head, too hard. I visited him a lot in the hospital. He was always asleep. I was sleepy, too, because I was pregnant with you. When you are pregnant you feel sleepy. All the time, sleepy. You also feel sleepy when you are sick, and Abu Fernando was sick. I would sleep with Abu Fernando, in the couch in his hospital room, like I slept in the couch in your hospital room, where we were last week.

I was very sad. Abu Fernando is my daddy, and in a way, he was gone. Alive but gone. Like you see him now. You were in my belly when I was very sad. Maybe you felt my sadness. But this sadness is not your sadness. It is mine. It is mommy's, not yours. You can be very, very happy even if mommy is sad. Sometimes, this is hard to know. But you must know it.

I was not sad for very long. Because even though my daddy was gone, you came, you were born. And I was so happy. Happy forever. Like I am now, because you are here. Do you understand.

Yes. Tell me another story.

Okay. Let's see.

But a really only happy story.

I look at boy's daddy. In bed listening to boy's mommy try to fix his boy's brain via internalization of fact. Of only happy fact.

Boy's daddy knows what to tell—

I am going to tell you the story of McLaren, the racecar company. It is really only happy.

Boy and I listen to the only happy story of the fast, triumphant cars of McLaren. I do not remember story now: stories of

cars are not stories I know how to internalize. But I remember
the onset of fixed.

vs.

Give him the Keppra, the frothy neurologist says, *and if the seizures
go away, then we know they were seizures.*

    For one hospital moment, we consider this wise. Of course:
Keppra. So that we can know seizure as seizure as such. It is
tempting to know. Knowing now vs. later vs. ever.

vs.

Conjecture abounds on the origins of the word "Prufrock."
Some say the word "prude" fused with the word "frock"
because "The Love Song of J. Alfred Prufrock" is a poem about
a prude in frock. Some say nowhere. Some say somewhere.
Some say furniture store in T.S. Eliot's hometown, a place
named St. Louis, Missouri.

    Incidentally, *ancestry.com* says five of the five Prufrock
families living in the U.S. are in Missouri. Missouri seems real
world far, but in terms of longing seems unremarkable, seems
identified.

    To the question of Prufrock perhaps the answer, in the
lamplight, is simply a name.

    In the lamplight, downed by a little brown name!

vs.

Partial focal seizures, seizures that originate in one area of the
brain, may be presaged by an aura. Onset foretold. Auras are
manifold, manifest as any number of: déjà vu, sharp, explosive
emotions, metallic taste, inexplicable audible voices, nausea,

unpleasant smell, detachment. Then seizure. As in sudden drop in air pressure, then tornado. Aura as margin, as moment when this begins to become that, is nearly that, now, watch it, it is happening, here is where your former life intersects with that.

Boy does not have auras to warn him of seizures. But boy has seizures. This, the doctors all say. Between three to six per day. He leans back, grasps a wall, giggles. Five seconds each. A condition. A conditioned life. As in, you may live, but on one condition. The condition is seizure.

Unremarkable vs. idiopathic. Idiopathic vs. you.

vs.

Below, some, not all, of the side effects of Keppra (A.K.A. Levetiracetam!):

- drowsiness
- weakness
- infection
- loss of appetite
- stuffy nose
- tiredness
- dizziness

In children, there are more:

- accidental injury
- hostility
- anxiety

Medicated dizziness, with risk of accidental injury, infection, hostility, to replace non-disruptive, non-injurious, dizziness marked by laughter.

And how, then, shall I presume.

vs.

Our days vary from:

It's happening.
It's happening.
It's happening.

to:

It's happening.
It's happening.
It's happening.
It's happening.
It's happening.
It's happening.

per day.

vs.

Last year, I began seeing auras. My aura. Those of other people. But first, that of one woman. A professor. In front of white-board. After staring for two hours, staring beyond, but also toward, it emerged. It was yellow, green on its edge. I saw it for a while before I realized what I was seeing. Once I realized, realized and gazed, it, aura, was gone.

I had to learn how to see, what I now knew how to see. Online, some tips: stare soft, stare fuzzy, stare beyond, stare unfocused. Stare off. Wait. Practice with own hand, between fingers of own hand, while hand is held above pliant white sheet, best time is post dawn.

I did not look up: aura is what. Incidentally, I knew. Aura is the during, to which the before is body, to which the after is world. Real world. The intersection of body's idea of life with body's actual life. Aura is indication, to which the seizure is world.

vs.

According to *St. Louis Magazine*, the name "Prufrock" would have denoted normalcy in the St. Louis of 1910. It would seem the idea of average averaged its way into the poem.

vs.

Whom to call when sad. Who. Who, who won't respond with compassion delivered as another's emotional load, with questions of procedure, questions of doubt, questions to which the answer is name, name I do not have, name of which the not having is so bad. Bad that becomes silence and breathing instead of voice on the line.

No, let's not do that. What is it I want. I want to dial a combination of ten numbers, a voice, familiar, to say: *It will be fine because you are good.* Then done, so long. I do not know correct combination to dial. I seek what I know I can find. Coffee, good and fine.

I sip the coffee. Open laptop. Select email to respond. My fingers press correct combination of keys. Press send. Sip. Sent. I know the names of words to use to respond. I feel it, the day-to-day onset of fine.

Of how am I. Why, thanks for asking, I am fine.

vs.

To say epilepsy is to say fever, the White Doctor says, *"epilepsy" is a blanket term for two or more unexplained seizures. Fever can be caused by a number of things, so can epilepsy. In many cases, the cause remains ignored.*

It is clear what White Doctor likes to say. Say little, say clear.

I read, I say, *that kids grow out of them. I read that some seizures go away.*

That is something I really cannot say.

No use to ask again, ask anything again, not even with words that sound different even when they are asking the same.

vs.

I write Elsa, the queen, queen doctor witch of Bogotá. Boy had six episodes yesterday, six more today, I write. Gluten, sugar, dairy, all gone. Nothing that lives in the sea. No electronics held by hand. Ten days since hospital. Nothing has changed.

The last time Elsa and I spoke was a day after our hospital discharge when I asked if this could be a case of Hamer points.

No, not your boy. He cannot be fixed by story, no matter how happy, no matter how deeply absorbed. Look up "le petit mal." What he has is physical, mercury hidden in layers of brain, perhaps, even from birth. There is real work for us to commence. For now, stay firm: no sugar, no dairy, no gluten, nothing at all that lives in the sea.

She also mentions Cuban doctor who lives in Guayaquil in whose possession a Russian magnetic machine. *Bring boy to me, but also to him. Consider a trip to Guayaquil. I fear, not diet alone. Connections of brain must be redrawn.*

They, the seizures, if seizures, are mild, I say.

Yes, says Elsa, *but they are frequent. Frequent is not a form of mild.*

She emails an order for more tests. More blood drawn from

within body of boy out into world to help draw this story of mystery, of mercury, perhaps, concealed inside boy, remarkable boy, day by day, redrawn.

Tráemelo.

vs.

A Hamer point: an area of darkness in brain generated by trauma that affects body based on spot where shock is processed. Boy has something more, more solid than shadow of trauma.

The story of Hamer points: German doctor Ryke Geerd Hamer's beloved boy is accidentally killed in 1978. Months later, Dr. Hamer is diagnosed with testicular cancer. Dr. Hamer feels certain his cancer is caused by death of beloved boy. He observes thousands of brains of patients with cancer, seeing shadows in brain, seeing patterns in the shadows in brain.

Same location of shadow for same type of cancer. Same type of conflict, of unresolved emotional issue, for same type of cancer. Knowledge that organs are linked to specific emotions is not new. Acupuncture practice applies this fact well.

What Dr. Hamer says that is new is this: each unresolved emotion eventually affects specific area of brain, each particular area of brain links to particular organ that unresolved emotion will in turn physically affect. Organ where cancer will sprout. Area of brain that is affected will darken, an observable dark point. A Hamer point. Cancer as psychosomatic disease. Cure as closure, as conflict focused, brought forth, so as to resolve. So as to heal.

My question is this: boy has epilepsy. Okay. Epilepsy is disease, disorder of brain. What is the emotion linked to sickness of brain. Are not all emotions, ultimately, declared by the brain. If so, then is disease of brain the somatic result of generalized ache.

vs.

Incidentally, the events of this story, all, so far, occur within a Mercury retrograde span. Of course, planets don't slow. It only appears to be so when Mercury travels in a direction opposed.

vs.

I close no doors, descend all rabbit holes. Roll toward the over-whelming question. Continue to ask: *what is it*. Sergio's pre-scription of life retold, new and improved, so that generational pattern is purged, not eternally foretold. The happy story of *mami*, of mom, of imagined maternal archetype, spoken to boy in bed, enfolded by the slim weight of thin cotton sheet—

When Abuelo Fernando did not wake up as himself, we were all very sad. It was a new day-to-day life. It was hard, this new life, especially for Abuela Ani. Remember, he used to walk, talk, remember names. Because it was so hard, Abuela was not happy.

Sometimes, when we are not happy, we can be mean. It is dif-ficult, when we are sad, to be good. Like when you are in trouble and can't watch TV, you yell, kick. Like this, Abuela yelled and she kicked, because it was like she could never again watch TV. Because I was always there, when she yelled and when she kicked, she yelled and she kicked at me. So, I was sad. Sad because Abuelo was no longer himself, sad for Abuela, sad to get kicked so often and so hard.

But even though this sounds like I had a lot of sad inside. I did not. Not everywhere. You were born. And your daddy and I were so happy. Happy not sad. Happy on top, sad on the bottom. Happy because of you.

This can happen, sad and happy at once. Happy can win, but we have to help it. We have to declare it. Like this: I am happy because of boy. Because of boy, because of his daddy, because of me, because my mind can say, this is good.

I was sad Abuela could not watch TV. *But, I had to learn it was her sad. Not my sad. I could still watch* TV. *Like this, you must learn my sad is never your sad. You don't need to be sad because mami is sad. Or papi. Mami and papi don't need to be sad if you are sad. Everyone's sad is their own sad. Sad is not a toy that you need to share to behave. It is good to be happy. Even if mami is sad. It is important to be good. Even if mami is sad. Do you understand?*

Yes. Tell me another story.

Ok.

An only happy story.

This time I am prepared with the story of Messi, Lionel Messi. Boy's beloved soccer idol. Story boy thinks he knows. But I am equipped.

Remarkable new details emerge.

vs.

I realize I am okay with sad. Sad as it once was, as it once meant. But I can only be sad alone. To darken, jagged and massive, alone. Sad about one single thing, sad because. Not sad as home. I am sad about seizure of boy. Sad about fresh fear we must learn to wield. Sad that seizures remain of cause unknown. Sad to consider changes to life seizure implies for boy. But reasons for sad are, as poet Claudia Rankine writes, dignified. Trustworthy. Real.

vs.

Friend of friend of friend's neurologist friend, recommends we consult cardiologist.

Episodes of boy don't sound like seizures, neurologist friend says. *If there is seizure, seizure must show on* EEG. *Clear* EEG *cannot be seizure. Check his heart. Dysrhythmia. Arrhythmia.*

Boy's grandfather has heart arrhythmia, I say. *We told doctors this at the hospital. They checked boy's heart. They performed an* EKG.

But during one of boy's episodes, neurologist friend asks.

No, not during.

If episode didn't happen while boy was hooked up to EKG, *nothing will register on* EKG. EEG, *like* EKG, *only records organic real-time. Get a Holter monitor, portable* EKG *machine, have them measure boy's heart for twenty-four hours. Episodes happen every day, correct.*

Yes, every day, several times, each day.

Good, that is good, neurologist friend says. *For our purposes, that is good.*

vs.

In car, as we leave hospital at the precise end of our hospital stay, Lucila calls. From the deep, from within the deep death of her Venezuela, she calls. What do doctors say.

Epilepsy, I say.

What did doctors give.

Keppra, I say.

Do not give boy Keppra. Esperen. And, when I return, bring boy to me. Tráemelo.

vs.

On Monday after MRI, before results are in, friend calls. *How is boy.*

Boy is fine. Episodes despite. CT *Scan clear.* EEG *clear.*

Why then need for MRI.

Better pictures. Clearer slices of brain. I think boy has a condition we will figure out how to treat.

But is that what doctors think.

No, I say, *that is what I think. It is what I say. Doctors don't say.*

I make note, silently, of what questions never to ask parent in hospital waiting for exams of child, make note, privately, of what words not to use that sound out loud.

vs.

On Monday after MRI, after results are in and, again, I am able to read, I begin reading second book brought. Clarice Lispector's *Near to the Wild Heart.* A book recommended by my friend Jonathan a few weeks before he died, sudden, unexpected. This is simply fact: a sad fact. It is sad to read the last book this friend will recommend, but the book is good, life while reading the book is good, too. I am happy, more than sad, to read the good book my friend Jonathan wanted me to read because he wished for me to be engulfed.

Novel is about a girl, Joana. When Joana is young, she asks her teacher what happens when a person becomes happy. To this, a perplexed teacher doesn't know quite what to respond. Joana, of course, insists. She wants to know: "being happy is for what?"

3

A week or so after hospital, I take boy to pediatrician. Pediatrician needs an update. Her records need an update.

Epilepsy, I say. *Keppra*, I say.

How's he doing with the Keppra.

We haven't administered yet.

Are you going to.

No, seizures are so mild. All he does is laugh, lean back. Keppra seems worse.

That's fine, I've had lots of kids whose seizures go away. I see your MRI cites possibility of dysplasia. Bear in mind my dysplasia kids tend to become my ADHD kids. Save the medicating for the ADHD.

He does not have ADHD. Anyway, I would not medicate.

No mom wants to medicate. Sometimes you have to. Kids have no friends, fall behind in school. Moms come here begging for it. Same moms who said they would never medicate. Meanwhile, give him CBD, but the very good kind, the kind with concentrated TCH. I'll call the pharmacy, let them know you're going. Explain the situation, the kind of thing you need.

Okay, I say. *Also, I want boy to bring own lunch to school. For this, I require a doctor's note.*

vs.

Eliot, repeatedly asked about the origin of the name *Prufrock*, wrote a letter in 1950 to acknowledge that perhaps he *was* aware of the name, somewhere deep within his mind. The Prufrocks were furniture dealers in his hometown, he later, post-poem, came to realize.

Name, internalized as fact, incidentally emerged.

vs.

I begin a Notepad entry on my phone with occurrence of epi-sodes. I name it *Frequency*—

3/8.	2
3/9.	1
3/10.	3
3/11.	3
3/12.	1
3/13.	2. Organic Rice Krispies
3/14.	3
3/15.	4. Holter monitor.
3/16.	6
3/17.	6. Vegan spirulina ice cream. No coco water.
3/18.	1. Bogotá
3/19.	2
3/20.	1. Bad night, at least 2
3/21.	3. Bad night, at least 2
3/22.	3
3/23.	6. Vegan gluten free chocolate muffin. Two
3/24.	3
3/25.	2

I wonder if boy ever really has one episode, or two. How well he reports, unknown. I believe if I keep good notes, I will figure boy's epilepsy out.

Do I.

vs.

What you get when you are happy is feeling good. But can sad be good. The "wakeful anguish" of which John Keats speaks in his '*Ode on Melancholy.*'

Sad, happy, good, bad: simple situations of mind, of brain. Brain that seizes, idiopathically, is bad, not good, sad, not happy. Is it.

What has changed. Boy is boy, with seizure of brain. At school, in car, at home. By sudden laughter seized. Do I feel sad. Do I.

Do I feel sad or just different. Can I name what I feel. Can I catalogue any of it. When I stand to walk away, when I pick up and hang up a call, when I sweat, when I bathe, when I select a menu plate, when I close the laptop for the day, what specifically can I say has changed.

vs.

Did they look for café con leche marks, my friend asks.

Yes, I say, *they found three. One on thigh, two on back. Did your boy have them.*

No. His seizures were horrible though. Like Poltergeist seizures. He had four.

Did they ever offer medication.

No. Doctors thought it was febrile seizures, and those go away. Get genetic testing. Insist on it. Genetic testing came close, closest, to telling us finally what Lionel had finally had.

vs.

Cuban doctor, Russian machine. Does the answer to the question lie flat on a plastic cot in the equatorial city of Guayaquil.

Is the answer to what a question of where.

vs.

At cardiologist's boy farts a lot. Boy farts smell adult toxic. It is only later that I consider having asked if this could be a symptom. I ask husband, worried I missed my chance to bring such important matters up. He tells me it is the vitamins, all the vitamins we are giving. All the vitamins boy is taking, eager to take. Vitamin B wafer, last left standing quarter-sized sweet delicacy.

At cardiologist's boy has episode. Cardiologist takes pulse, eager to rule out heart, signal the brain. As if cardiologist defending organ of heart. Good ol' heart would never do that. Oh no, that's the brain, typical brain effed up shit behavior.

I have no problem installing a Holter monitor, but this is not the heart, cardiologist says.

I say, yes-please-yes. Install monitor of heart.

Boy leaves with cables and tape attached. I am happy— or, am I a happy mom.

Talk of symptomatic farts in car ride home funny enough to laugh.

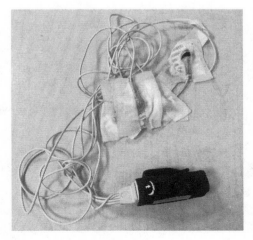

vs.

I return to Lispector, move slowly, push, pry, fingers pliant to the edges, eager to allow its eager taking. It is dense, but there are openings, too. As vision the experience could be named "tangled mangrove root."

Book is about a girl named Joana. My friend who recommended it, Jonathan. Jonathan before he dies. Unfortunate mixture of substance inserted. Wrong combination of fun.

Jonathan/Ana. Jo/Ana. Joana.

I notice this right combination of name/s on a night I strain to read because life is sad because of death of friend, seizure of boy. But just normal sad. Stupid death. Mild seizure. Bothered by it all. Day in, day out.

When I call Jonathan's mother to share grief, I tell her I'm annoyed at Jonathan. Like if he was still there to receive, to deflect, to formulate excuse for senseless combination of fun.

She laughs, an acute, shrill laugh. A brief laugh. *It's true*, she says. *I'm annoyed, too*. I laugh back, brisk, brusque, brute, we laugh.

It would feel good to brew her good coffee. Show her how my good coffee trick shepherds the onset of fine. But she lives somewhere unreachably far.

vs.

It is happening:
Boy laughs.
Mother snaps.
Sums the seconds, counts
The bouts.
It's not over:

                        But,
            It
            Stopped.

vs.

Six or more *café con leche* marks are diagnostic tool for neuro-fibromatosis. A genetic disorder that can be very bad. I don't bother reading more. My boy has three: three marks from birth. Not six or more. The internet is very specific about six or more.

Fine vs. five vs. more.

Genetic is not idiopathic. It is genetic because humans know what gene, exactly, when mutated causes disease. When doctors know gene, they say they know what is medical, clinical cause. Cause is gene. Gene is cause.

But gene knowledge seems to me a mere assurance of location, of symptomatic source. Wherefrom a flaw built-in, emerges. A place with a name on a map, not an understanding of such place, much less of source. Place from whence onset transpires.

Yet is gene a why. Is it a what. Is it, deeply, a how.[2]

Heretofore, mother's and father's DNA combine to form boy. But, how does body know what or how to grow. And why, why form this one specific right combination of life. Mother is granted a belly of boy. Substance inserted, live birth, out comes boy with flaw imbedded since first cell formed. Seizure, henceforth.

White Doctor says only seventy percent of human genome mapped. Also, only fifty percent of seizures have genetic

---

2   No. It is not.

marker presented as cause. This does not mean thirty percent of unmapped genome, when mapped, will give name to fifty percent of idiopathic seizures.

The White Doctor only states what he knows. He knows to be careful. Genetic is tempting. Temptation of answer. Statistic of solve. He says, *Let's do the testing but be warned of how little we know.*

vs.

I've entered the domain of disease. When you enter you learn what outlandish words mean. You need these words because of "it." To approach "it," you must operate words others have assembled to encircle disease.

vs.

Days after hospital I go to Nelly, beloved local Reiki worker, who mixes formula for premature babies at hospital where we were with boy, whom we saw at hospital with boy, who has written me many times post-hospital.

Come see me, she says, *I will wipe the hospital off. Reiki dispels the memory that lingers, malingers, off. Off from aura of body of soul.*

I do as all my witches say. Go in, lie down, command open my centers to foreign open hands. Nelly begins. Usually, we are quiet; this time she speaks.

Get him tested for Epstein-Barr virus, she says. *Most of this country has it. But if he has it, you have to get rid of it. Causes all forms of havoc. You can eliminate it via diet.*

Tell me more, I say

I have breast cancer, she says. I did not know. She tells me more, about her sickness and how she is healing through food. No sugar, no dairy, no wheat, fully vegan.

I will check him, Nelly, I say, and mean it because what Nelly says during Reiki, I do. *Tell me,* I say, *why is this happening, what is the larger lesson here, for me.*

It is your poetry, believe it or not. In part, this is happening because you must focus on your poetry, believe it or not.

I believe it, I say, and she believes me because I am unsurprised.

vs.

Name boy gives episodes is "Messi," name of beloved soccer player legend. It is the code word boy will use to tell his teacher, a former professional figure skater who keeps sugar-free lollipops in her desk drawers, that "it" is happening. Code word: Messi. "Messi," "it" is.

How many Messis did you have at school.

Zero, Mimi. Zero.

Mimi: code word for me.

But, once boy is home from school, at least three. Almost every day, after school, at least three. Around four, around seven, in bed, right before sleep. In the notepad entry *Frequency,* I continue to keep count. Continue to mull over what happens to boy when I am not around.

vs.

In Jonathan's Lispector, remarkable Joana refers to herself in the third person to allow herself wider thoughts.

From reading Jonathan's Lispector, Ana remarks—

I, too, can change pronouns when I write, like Lispector. "I" can become "she" so as to abstract my thoughts from myself, cast them wider. Wider as in looser, not so tight-fitting, my thoughts. Easier to fathom because more wind beneath wingspan of thought.

Mother-arc-thoughts spring for answers to questions of boy with episodes, named "seizures" by doctors. But I seek to name with a more complete combination of words. She, Ana, realizes that her search will need to be ampler, sundry, so as to snare name in the tapered medical jurisdiction of idiopathic-sounding jargon.

To ask what is it. To ask it silently, within. And from within generate action without. Action unannounced, private. So as to avoid feelings of sad, which are mild, tolerable, in private. She realizes this. Ana realizes this. Sadness, for her, does not happen while alone. I am mentally a workhorse, I think. I demand for myself to be stable, to be firm. I am a smooth wooden tool, she says. Splinterless. Deliberate as toil, gravid as soil. Both action and element plied by control.

Furthermore, Jonathan lives, I reckon. Yet, Jonathan passed, Ana thinks. I can reckon what Ana cannot think.

Boy walks up and says, *why are you writing Mimi.*

(Interruption!) (Lamplight!)

Because I like to read and write. That's what I like to do.

Why did you write, "Jonathan passed, Ana thinks," boy who can recently read asks.

Because that is what I think, and I write what I think.

Take out the part that says "Ana thinks."

Why.

Because then everyone will know what the whole story is about.

vs.

This picture is a picture of Jonathan who somehow was, who somehow no longer is:

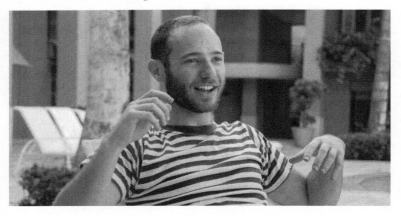

vs.

Soy sauce has wheat.
   Vitamins have sugar.
      Seizures accrete.
         The question is not   what.
Not
   what is
   it.
   The question is   can you live
   with   it.
The question is   when you
         sit
   and think
      how bad really   is
      it.

vs.

The color of your aura changes depending on how, what, why you are presently living life. If you are living mostly from a spiritual growth pursuit then your aura is lavender. If you are living from an absorbing dynamic activity pursuit, then your aura is yellow. Or yellow green. If your life is passion, vigor, energy then aura is red. Duh. Red is fire, since the beginning, red always means blaze.

Auras can change. This I find important. Important in that I can see auras so I can see changes manifest in real world. Clues. Perhaps, clues of boy, of what is within boy.

Aura information is readily available within internet, mostly found in poorly designed websites because hokey pokey has regrettable graphics. Why can't hokey pokey aura color design be crisp. Chakra pictures modern, sleek, like an ad for a co-working space that serves turmeric matcha oat lattes. Srsly.

Hokey pokey deserves better design. Once idea is in my mind, I want to say it out loud. But to whom. Who could be this whom. Instead, I write idea down. Like this, within becomes without.

Boy's aura is yellow, consistently. Not yellow versus anything. Yellow. A constant of free, fun-loving energy. Mine was lavender before unremarkable laughter of idiopathic seizure began. Now I see it as blue, very pale, wan blue. Like the core of a lit Zippo lighter. Blue is associated with healing. Lavender with spirit, fantasy. I've checked to be sure many times it is blue. It remains blue, blue like the color of focused gas fire.

vs.

To get a second opinion you must first get medical records of first opinion. This is wicked. What is wicked is this:

obtaining medical records, really it is. Literally, accurately bad.
Unadulteratedly bad. Non-source-plumbing experience of bad
with no taking to be had. Entire hours on hold. Recordings
that were recorded to explain what letters to mail in order to
retrieve records by mail. Meanwhile, the records are yours,
a latent key to your health. Press one to hear this recording
again. One is the only option. Look for pen paper press one
write down address by hand. Nowhere an email address. Where
do you want your records faxed. Faxed. You can also fax your
request over. Fax. If you do not have fax you can come here and
drop off then return to pick up. Come here. First drop off, then
come back and pick your records up. Or fax. When you fax
include description of your illness but not the doctor version
but description written in your own words. If patient is minor
then describe that happens to patient in your own words. Also,
your relation to minor. I am mother of boy. Do your records
not show that. Exercise in humility. Humility of she who has
the pen and paper in hand, pen and paper to take down number
of fax. Or address to go because fax. Fax. Please do not forget
to include cover letter for your fax. Please remember to include
your information your relation to boy your contact information what records you require if not all in the cover letter which
presents your request for the records of your boy. Via fax. Can
you email anything. Can you confirm receipt. No. No, no this
is not funny in the moment of living. But funny because ridic-
ulous in the reading. I mean. I want control over documents
to send out. I want to own information of boy, boy who the
country's laws deem my own. My boy is my boy is not your
boy medical record recording sir. Dear sirs, attached to this
letter please find my request for the records you hold for my

boy. The record of his examinations, I want them all: all of the incidental and non-incidental findings as a result of any and all examinations, records of his diagnosis, even if they proclaim idiopathic epilepsy.

O, release my records, boy's records, to me, guardian, mother of boy, kind, wise, dear sirs.

vs.

"Fax," I decide, is an appropriate word for situations that require the usage of "fuck."

What the fax.

vs.

I have premonition of onset of darkness in New Jersey while visiting friend who is there for radiation treatment for her baby. Baby Anaya. Premonition happens while I am there, two weeks before boy is admitted to hospital. Of course, premonition is impossible to prove. Seldom is it shared. Rarely, even as matter of retrospect, conversed.

To clarify, premonition is not New Jersey's fault. As previously discussed, New Jersey as candidly temporary location is not flawed.

Premonition is linked to pattern. I recognize a pattern in my being in New Jersey, visiting friend in need of help. A pattern in my being away from my own children, own home. The pattern here is this: woman with healthy children visits woman who needs help with children before healthy children of visiting woman become unwell.

Of course, pattern is pattern because it already happened. At least once. And so, it has. Pattern begins with other friend, mother to Lionel, who visits a mother who needs help with children days before Lionel passes.

Mother to Lionel had premonition and shares premonition with me. Privately, in retrospect, shares. If not for this uncharacteristic sharing I perhaps would not have recognized own premonition. Own premonition in own mind is mere specter of shadow. There is no rattle of skeleton. It is a nudge, a haze from which no material motion emerges. The muffled non-recognition of paler recognition.

Because premonitions happen so deep within mind, so deep within brain, premonitions work so well within books. As reader, you know things characters do not say, do not formulate. The writer coolly slips perception in so that you, as reader, can know.

Except here there is nothing more I as writer can coolly slip. You and I, word by word, we advance together: we are on the same page.

vs.

I, like boy, am no better than myself.

vs.

Dramamine. The pediatrician gives us Dramamine. I give boy Dramamine. Boy takes kids' Dramamine. Purple pellet designed to taste sweet.

It feels good to say Dramamine. Innocent as in before.

vs.

In my own words, here is how I am able to understand the following:

a. Gliosis—a swelling, rearranging, reprograming of glial cells
    in the brain. Glial cells and neurons are the two types of cells
    in brain. Glial cells live between neurons and protect them.
    There are many types of glial cells, such as astrocytes, oligo-
    dendrocytes, ependymal cells, Schwann cells, satellite cells
    and microglia. When glial cells are hurt, for example, soccer
    ball smash to the head, something similar to scarring results.
    "Gliosis" is the name by which doctors convey scar.
b. Hypomyelination—this means low myelination. Myelin-
    ation is fat around the nerve cells that is necessary for cells to
    work like they need to work. Absence of fat around nerves.
    Starvation.
c. Dysplasia—this explanation is courtesy of super friendly
    doctor in hospital who tells us that she would not have
    reported any marking on boy's MRI. She explains dysplasia
    as an event that happens in utero an instant of confused,
    anarchic, wild brain cell growth. The instantaneous dis-
    order of cellular growth leaves a smudge visible on MRI.
    The name with which doctors trap the smudge is dysplasia.
    Because skin and brain form at same congenital time, birth-
    mark of skin can indicate birthmark of brain. Dysplasia.
    This is the type of smudge, of mark, that Elsa says Cuban
    doctor in Guayaquil can fix. With a lot of oxygen, with
    magnets. With trip to Guayaquil—fix.

In terms of contrast, here is how the previous terms interact:

Bruise vs. Emaciation vs. Birthmark

In terms of severity, here is how the latter terms associate:

Gliosis = Hypomyelination = Dysplasia

In terms of magnetic resonance imaging of brain, I am unable to say how they, the three remarkable manifestations of imperfection of brain, can appear to be one and exactly the same.

One vs. all; all vs. any; any vs. none; versus vs. nothing whatsoever at all.

vs.

I call my friend, mother to Lionel, after watching a Barcelona soccer game with boy.

I just learned the coolest thing, I say. *Do you know what Messi's first name is?*

Um, yeah. Lionel. That's who we named Lionel after.

What. Really. How did you ever even watch Messi.

I don't know, she says. *I guess it was the World Cup. Everyone watched a little of that. I saw his name on the screen and thought it was a cool name. Who'd you think I named him after. Not Lionel Ritchie.*

I laugh. *Yes. Well, no, not after Lionel Ritchie. Like not in honor of him, although Lionel Ritchie is no doubt awesome. But just that you'd seen the name there.*

My friend laughs. We laugh together. Comfortable and capacious. Natural, we laugh.

vs.

It's easy to live in present moment of child when there is fear for future of child. Once there is fear for future of child present becomes absence of future.

I'll explain:

a. There is talk at a table of children as adolescents. What will my child be like, yours, theirs. I cannot imagine child as future child anymore. Child is only child today because of—what if. Because of—what will happen. Because of—what is happening. I cannot imagine boy tomorrow. Boy is only boy now.

b. Plans for summer grow difficult, different. Will there be swimming. Boy should not. And if boy does not swim should boy not attend camp. Will boy be weird. Let's not go there yet. Let's just stay here.

c. It is happening happens in front of other kids. So far, kids are little, they don't really stop and think. When do kids stop and think. Around second grade, in two years. Will we need to medicate then. Will seizures be gone then. Will we have to talk to kids in school then. Will kids be cool. Will they be awful. Mean. Of course, yes, of course there will be a mean kid or two. Do we wait to think about these things until right before, right before the moment when kids stop to start to think. Yes. Let's.

For now, let's remain here, let's remain now. What is happening is only happening now.

vs.

Cardiologist is right. Whatever boy has, it is not a *mal* derived from material organ of heart. Heart is good, unremarkably good. Boy's circulation of blood is fine. But the brain, oh, the brain, typical brain effed up idiopathic shit behavior.

Boy is fine, the hospital doctors say. Mild, frequent seizure of brain is a thing, a moment, an incident, that is not life-threatening, that is within the feasible realm of fine. Seizures don't do anything to body. It's what happens during seizures, while boy goes through life, the hospital doctors say, that poses risk to life. Seizure, in and of itself, is fine.

But how to separate seizure, in and of itself, from life.

vs.

With husband in car, with husband in bed, with husband on phone, with husband at work, with husband at coffee, we talk, we text, of boy. With husband anywhere we talk about boy. Is it getting better. Worse. Same. Same is worse. Or is same better. Same does not feel like same. Same feels like worse. Except we read about breadth of seizure in real world and same feels like better. Until, again, it feels like worse.

My phone rings.

A call from Lithuania, I say to husband. Move my hands so as to hang up junk call on the screen of my phone. Another tele-marketer call. Sale of pain killers, insulin, healthcare.

Give it to me, Nelson David takes phone from my hands.

He answers call.

You are the scum of the world, he says, yells. *The worst. Worst in the world.*

The person who called from a place called Lithuania hangs up.

I look at husband.

You should try it, he says. *It really helps. Works great, actually.*

Okay, I say, *next time, I'll yell.*

vs.

Boy as filter, boy as other, boy as same, same as mother, as father. Boy as filter, at once, of all that is part, of all that is other.

Boy as filter. Of that which blends but also of that which sets far, further along, farther apart.

vs.

In telling others what pediatrician says about her dysplasia/sei-zure kids, about saving the medicating for when boy later gets ADHD, I come crawling to realize:

I liked hearing pediatrician say what she says about seizure kids becoming ADHD kids, but others do not and are shocked because it is a horrible thing to hear. Save your medicating for when boy has ADHD is a horrible thing to say because it is a hor-rible thing to hear.

I admit: I agree: the content of the statement terrible. But I know from sitting in a room with pediatrician and hearing her speak that what she says is said because it is true. It is not wicked of her to narrate a story many times true. Factually, her dys-plasia/seizure kids become her ADHD kids. Sure, no mother wants to medicate. But, certainly, mothers flock to her des-perate to medicate.

It is not bad that pediatrician says this. What is bad is not affair of her statement. What is bad is hard truth. The story, many times lived, many times told, many times true. A real-world fact that dysplasia has no solution other than medication now or medication later.

But I liked hearing her speak, liked the sound of the voice of a doctor who delivers hard truth.

I realize , too, that pediatrician never asks what kid eats. What kid does. Who kid is. How mom moms. How dad dads. There are no questions. There is diagnosis. Diagnosis leads to prognosis. Prognosis is good because medication takes away symptoms that prompt diagnosis. Like going back in time to before, to before *it is happening*. When nothing happens there is nothing to see, to seize, here.

Prognosis is condition controlled, disease suppressed. Administer medication. Seizure goes. Normal returns. Now or later. If later, then seizure will continue, elongate. Live with seizure, adapt to seizure, scrutinize seizure, or medicate.

Keppra, the Keppra, our Keppra, sits quiet as closed cabinet in the husk of a vacant home.

vs.

At some point during this, during the *it's happening* of this. During the writing and the living of this. I stop praying.

I pray a lot. Usually, I pray a lot. It is a private form of prayer that does not involve congregational mediation. It is probably similar to meditation. To cushion of silence. To abstraction. To immersion into secret life. To absconding from day before day starts and breaking away, again, prior to sleep of night. My prayer is probably too simple. Too simple to fill vaulted, gothic air, too simple to tally as denominational.

Prayer, too, happens in car. It happens in bed. It happens while reading to boy. It happens after each and every doctor's visit where I think thank God boy gets to go to doctor. Even if it is a fight with boy to get boy to doctor. Even if doctor gives not answer, not proposed solution, not sign, not promise, not optimism, not progress.

Then, prayer stops. Is it me who stops prayer. Me or my exhaustion. Me or my anxious undertow of fear. What within me. Conclusions derived from experience come slow. It takes me weeks to acknowledge prayer stops. Weeks to realize it's been weeks. To ask myself, to pause, to enshroud silence, to focus, to abstract from life to be able to posit a why.

Absence of prayer is a ceasing of interrogation. Absence of prayer is not question but unquestionable faith. In the morning, in the evening, no longer in stillness, do I perform full-frontal beseeching, begging, of God. Because I don't pray, I don't ask, I don't question. I don't doubt.

Deliverance is in the deliberate way I ignite my car. In the way I brake for red. Brake because it is not my turn, not yet, to cross. In my wait, in my sufficient pressure applied to pedal of brake, is prayer.

Absence of prayer. Deficiency of doubt.

Prayer in crisis evolves: entire transient body becomes day-to-day, real-world manifestation of ask: God please help me name what it is and please let the name not command death.

I do not pray within, pray before, pray upon, pray to prep the movements of day. I do not drink hot water with lemon upon the first sight of day. I do not pause before good coffee served by thick ceramic pot. Perform none of the rituals I performed before onset of seizure of small six-year-old boy.

I feel I do not require them: the rituals, the rites. Feel this for a while without stopping to acknowledge such thought. Sense without saying. In crisis: unremarkable hum, inconspicuous chant. In crisis, survival.

I believe God does not require my ritual of bent knee because now I am prostrate even when standing—already bent on both knees. I trust God knows I beg for onset of seizure of boy to be contained, like coin in palm of closed hand, clasped.

This is the faith I believe.

vs.

Is writing a form of aura.

A symptom, a convulsion, a pervious membrane, the materialization, the crust of within intersected by without. Birthmark-like.

vs.

Scripted stage directions for seizure as scenic theater:

From stage left, enters running boy with soccer ball. Face flushed.

Enters kitchen. Well lit, clean. Woman in kitchen, presumably, boy's mother.

Boy: Mami, Mimi, I want coconut water.

Mami, Mimi: How do you say.

Boy: Mimi may I have some coconut water please.

Mami, Mimi: Of course.

Mami, Mimi opens fridge and pulls out container with, presumably, coconut water while boy waits beside her.

While Mami, Mimi opens fridge boy begins to walk backward from beside woman to kitchen cabinets next to fridge. Leans back against cabinets, head bent forward in forty-five-degree angle, upper back caved in, as if someone, something, tickling where neck meets the spine. Left arm bent up in ninety-degree angle, stiff, hand half-open, as if holding invisible glass. Boy giggles, laughs.

Mami, Mimi immediately steps back from fridge. Looks at boy. For three seconds she is whispering as if counting seconds inside her head, stares at boy as if waiting to spring should she need to break boy's fall. Closes fridge. Two more seconds pass. Mami continues to mouth a count.

Boy: It stopped. Can I have some coconut water.

Mami, Mimi: Yes, here.

Mami, Mimi quickly serves boy coconut water. Boy quickly drinks coconut water, quickly grabs ball to go back, presumably, outside.

vs.

Fax.

vs.

Simultaneous to seizure is work, is operative logistics of life.
Fingers and wrists, all day, respond to the various imperative
matters at hand. The company I run is for sale. Getting ready for
sale is a lot of document spreadsheet work. A lot of arranging
meetings, a lot of phone calls, a lot of travel work. Also, lawsuit
my company filed is ready to settle. Lawsuit is ready to settle
because of Eli, Elizabeth, the good witch at the heart of my
Bogotá. Really, it is.

Get a man to talk to the guy whose company you are suing, she says.
*This guy will never settle with a woman. He is a guy who does not like
the fiber of women.*

So, I get Nelson David to talk to the guy whose company
I am suing. Husband Nelson David loves the job of talking to
the guy whose company I am suing. Loves intermediary, con-
ciliator role, the role of good guy trying to talk some sense into
wife to try and get her to settle but you don't know my wife
don't know how stubborn she is and she will never settle for that
so you better take offer back to your board, friend.

She is source of laughter for husband and I—she, the wife
who won't settle, will not, will never settle for less, for anything
less than that. She is me, but she is not me. The wife. That wife
whom you don't know, do not know what she is like. She is me,
the wife, me if I was not looking. But I am looking, looking
hard. Because I am the wife who looks, I laugh. Laugh at guy
who thinks he and husband are, in secret, sharing a laugh.

Husband teaches me how settling is fun because guy will
lose and it is a matter of waiting, but there are many ways in

which to wait. Not answering is a form of wait. Answering partially is another. Answering sufficiently then completely forgetting to respond to guy whose company I am suing, have been suing, for longer than twenty months.

With the right wait, husband says, *you will reach the right amount. In the meantime, this guy is a comedy, let's laugh.*

Eli, Elizabeth, beloved witch, is right. I tell her, too, so we, too, the fiber women, can laugh.

Weeks pass. Husband texts, transcribes the messages drafted by my female hand. Sends responses to our comic guy.

It is slow, this moving forward between guy, between woman and man who are husband and wife, who are mom and dad, who are tired of counting the episodes of their boy. Mom and dad perfect the wait: forget to respond to guy: seizures consume, they truly forget. Outmaneuver the amount.

Simultaneous to seizure is work. Anything, simultaneous to seizure, no matter how laughable, is work.

vs.

Take the Keppra, take the boy home.

vs.

Is medication a form of heal. Give the body what it needs, no.

vs.

It is my friend, mom of Lionel, who gives me *The Philosophy of Andy Warhol, From A to B and Back Again,* written by Andy Warhol, during our time living together in college. Five years of living together. This friend is a friend who is different from all friends. Witness of youth to adulthood friend.

There is a practicality to emotionality that I learned from her. As in stay away from emotionality. Keep it together. Keeping it together is good. Good like a walk in Brooklyn with light backpack is good.

Does absence of emotionality limit amplitude of joy, of sorrow. I ponder. I pause. I hope to understand clearly how I long to feel, and what. I focus the lamplight hard.

Am I sad. Is seizure of boy sad.

There are options. Keppra, diet, second opinions. MRI is basically clear. What is so bad. Seizure itself is laughter. A succinct leaning back. Fully conscious, a no-more-than-five-second lapse. Am I sad because it is my fault. The crap diet, electronic apparatus overload fault of before.

Is sentiment of sad a feeling of heart or a thought administered by mind. Is it of heart and mind combined. Nothing has changed. Boy scores goals at soccer practice just like before. I remind myself of gratitude, of thankfulness, because always there is worse.

Perhaps it is fear. Sadness now because new fear. Nostalgia for moment when we did not live with fear of seizure of boy, seizure that could get worse, seizure that does not improve, seizure of source unknown. I am sad for myself and for my husband who now encounter new fear. Sad, too, for boy, who encounters new limits.

But, because of practicality of emotionality, I do not sink. Aim at good, knowing that in the movement toward there already is good. Remind myself of worse. Summon belief that seizure is problem that husband and I will solve.

Or not. A problem we will not solve, not decipher. One we will resolve: a condition to manage without panic or absolute control. In my own words, the words that come are these: fact of the matter can become heart of the matter. Seizure is no laughing matter, but I can choose to say it's not a crying matter.

Come over. Seriously, come over. Watch our words form, words that take so as to become. Yes, overtake: yes, overcome.

4

The Lord hath created medicine out of the earth; and he that is wise will not abhor them. Ecclesiasticus 38:4, King James Version (KJV)

At night, each night, boy asks me to lie next to him until he falls asleep. He falls asleep in my bed. Even if he is with friends and ignores me all day, he wants me at night. He names it snuggle puff. Me he calls *Mimi*. Mimi, he says, *I want snuggle puff.* He also wants to chat: about science facts we read. Also, about soccer. I have to say, *I will snuggle puff but only if you go to sleep. Tomorrow there is school. I am not answering any more questions, it is time, you need to sleep.* Being firm like this, gentle like this, makes me feel like a good mom, or is it like a mom who is good.

vs.

For many years, I believed "lovesong" to be a word. But now I know I was wrong, though I still think "love" and "song" belong together as one.

About where T.S. Eliot got the idea for the title of the Prufrock poem there is clarity. From Rudyard Kipling's poem "The Love Song of Har Dyal."

Har Dyal was a man whose full name was Lala Har Dyal. He was a rebel Indian Nationalist, rebelling against the British, decades before Gandhi. A sage, too, who wrote books on Buddhism and education, the most famous *Hints for Self Culture.* Har Dyal died in Philadelphia in 1939, hours after having lectured on this book.

Kipling was a fan of India at the time of Har Dyal. Eliot a fan of Kipling at the time Eliot was a young man alive. I a fan of

Eliot since the time I learned to private read and private write. It is in this remarkable way that Har Dyal and his "Beloved" enter my book, rectangular as chronology, in your upheld hands.

Come back to me, Beloved, or I die!

It is in this way that we get to be sad together, sad for Har Dyal (who is so miserable he will die!). Tell me it does not feel good to feel sad together for the long-gone man who, for an eternal poem instant, is so forlorn enough to die.

vs.

Spring Break in America. Time to take a national break from bad weather before our spirit breaks. Boy is on vacation. Things at work slow down. Let us go to Bogotá, we say. Let us go there, family and I.

Tráemelo, all the witch doctors say, bring boy to me.

vs.

Epstein-Barr virus test comes back positive. We look back, reconstruct. Switch the light of lamplight on. One month before onset of seizure, boy gets impetigo, skin infection caused by streptococcus and staphylococcus bacteria. Immediately during antibiotics for impetigo, boy with fever. At pediatrician, boy on antibiotics but with fever is tested and is negative for flu A/B. Fever gone. Boy still not himself. Call from school. Boy not himself. No fever, no mucus. No symptoms. Despite.

Epstein-Barr, the mononucleosis virus. The tired virus. The kissing bug. Boy had it a month before onset, concurrent with impetigo, four weeks before onset. Boy not himself between virus and onset, something must be within boy.

Could it be: virus vs. boy.

vs.

Incidentally, I discover experience of sadness of mind is identical to exhaustion at keeping shit together. Sadness as distinct desire for silence. For aloneness. For good coffee in silence. It is in this way that it is wholly possible to just be tired. And for that, theoretically, there is sleep, coffee. How am I. I am tired. I dispense good coffee. Now. Ask me again. How am I. What am I. Who.

I am someone who metes out good.

vs.

Boy has seizures in front of following medical practitioners (at time of writing):

- ER French Doctor
- White Doctor
- Cardiologist
- Sergio
- Doctor Carmona
- The Vet
- White Doctor (follow-up)
- White Doctor's assistant

Boy's doctor-available waking hours are from nine to five. Eight total hours. Eight hours times sixty minutes times sixty seconds totals 28,800 seconds and has some five episodes per day. Boy's episodes last five seconds.

Chances of doctor seeing an episode are:

$$\frac{25}{28,800}$$

Chances of seven doctors seeing an episode are:

$$\frac{5}{28,800} \times \frac{5}{28,800} \times \frac{5}{28,800} \times \frac{5}{28,800} \times \frac{5}{28,800} \times \frac{5}{28,800} \times \frac{5}{28,800} \times \frac{175}{201,600}$$

When working with probability, or chance, it is important to remember that the odds of one thing versus another require addition. But the chances of one thing and one more thing and yet one more of the same thing happening in summation result in multiplication. This is because it is harder for many of the same things to happen in a specific sequence of aggregate events than for one thing to happen versus another. Randomness is more likely than precise progression. Than specific sequence of events of life.

$$\frac{175}{201,600}$$

In a way, this number is the numerical expression of "it." Of what in God's name is it. Of *it is happening*. Of *it is happening* right now in front of a doctor.

Expressed as a reduced fraction, "it" looks like this:

$$\frac{7}{8064}$$

Articulated as decimal, *it is happening*, has happened, in front of a doctor seven times (at the time of writing) looks like this:

0.000868055555556

I wonder what, numerically, stoppage looks like. If *it has stopped* would be fraction, subtraction, negative mathematical expression. A sudden return to right from plunge into wrong combination of.

vs.

Nelly, beloved local Reiki worker who mixes formula for premature babies at hospital where we were with boy, whom we saw at hospital with boy, recommends a book for me to read, no not read, to listen to in audio form, the *Medical Medium*. *Don't read it,* she says*, because knowing you, you'll get bored. Download it and listen to it in traffic.*

My first audio book. Never before was I open to book in oracular form. Always before needing physical paper of literal book. But this is a time to let go of before. Before has something wrong. Something that, undisturbed, led to episode.

I hear book in car. It's written by guy Anthony Williams visited by a spirit being who tells him what other people have wrong, as in physically, literally wrong. Then Williams offers cures, cures of food and of herbs: blueberries, celery, onion, parsley, spinach, lemon balm, cat's claw. Medicine of only good food. Williams is better known as celery juice guy.

A few chapters into oracular book I visit www.medicalmedium.com because I am beginning to believe—and need to confirm validity via professional looking (AKA legit!) website.

There are many testimonials, including some by Sylvester Stallone, Naomi Campbell, major athletes, major CEOs, Robert De Niro. Others.

I keep listening. Interiorize while sitting still in traffic. Summarize story of boy to friends who ask about boy. Boy has episodes. Doctor prescribes Keppra. We resist, embark on search. Search leads to Nelly, leads to book. Confirmation of no dairy, no wheat, no sugar.

Give the body what it needs, no.

Behold as we immerse, drill the depth of portend, of bode. Behold us roll, not stroll, down every single rabbit hole.

Spirulina, cat's claw, marshmallow, celery, burdock, goldenseal roots. Cassandra conveyed within steel frame of car, oracle tows forth, forecast is audible, I shift into drive.

vs.

The worst thing you can call a Colombian is a Columbian. Any other name-calling related to historic heavy dark shit is, in some ways, anchored to fact. Fact we brush off.

But the term Columbian is based on total disregard for fact. Disregard as in lack of regard, as in do not give a shit. Dark shit is better than no shit. As in you better give a shit enough to get the name of nation right.

Colombia is not spelled Columbia. It's just not.

Perhaps, the confusion is understandable as "Columbus" in English is clearly not "Colombus." On the other hand, "Colón" in Spanish is clearly "Colón," not "Colún." What's more, English as language, as philology, grasps "colonize," "colony," "colonial" just fine.

There is no doubt what the name "Colón" looks like when harnessed against other.

Perhaps it is fitting—or is it fate—that a nation name set up to honor Columbus' repellant legacy be plagued by orthographical plunder.

vs.

In Colombia, I make appointments for boy to see Elsa, Sergio, Elizabeth. Not in that order. The actual order is Sergio, Elizabeth, Elsa.

Are we really going to go, husband asks. *Really go see all of them. All in one week.*

Yes, I say. *We are. We are really going to go see all of them with boy in one week. All of them. All will see boy.*

I am thrilled. I am thankful. I tell husband just you wait, soon, oh the happy days, soon, will come.

vs.

There is a little girl in this story of boy with sudden idiopathic seizure. His sister. Younger sister of boy with seizure is three. She is fine and good. Medically clinically unremarkable. Also funny. Too funny. Out of context funny in her home. Out of place, like sudden bout of seizing laughter.

But in place, holding place, fastening parents firm to place, to day-to-day, to within, to inside, to context of home, which she holds, beholds as setting of story with only happy end.

I watch her pretend to be a puppy. Asking me to invent a leash. *Are you real,* I say. She thinks question is real, so she gives real answer.

In her three-year-old stumble she says, *my face is real. I am Nina real.*

Nina, real.

It feels good to get this answer. I tie ribbon leash round puppy neck of Nina Real.

vs.

Some six weeks after we leave hospital, I stop updating *Frequency,* notepad entry with number of seizures per day, on my phone. Every day has become same, the same. Four to six Messis, episodes, seizures, remarkable idiopathic events each day.

All the supplements, changes in diet, result, really, in no change. No sugar, no gluten, no dairy. Magnesium, zinc, selenium, B-complex, probiotics, herbal immune drops.

Got boy to eat fruit. To put it in his mouth, chew, swallow. Not spit. Got him to eat all of following:

- Spinach, onion, tomato (blended as sauce)
- Broccoli
- Carrots
- Bananas
- Blueberries (with stevia sprinkled atop)
- Strawberries
- Apples
- Watermelon (highly occasional)
- Lemon
- Seaweed (made to look like salty thin chips)

No birthday parties, no casual outings, no going over to other children's houses, no access to electronic apparatus. Each and every meal at home for span of two months. Lunch box prepared for boy to eat at school.

Am asked if anything feels like progress. Boy is different, better, more well. Yes. Steadier. More tranquil. Even aware. I can state, boy is better. Boy is better, a phrase I am able to utter. But episodes, those, remain same. The same. Brief, non-disruptive, unsettling laughter four to six times per day. Every day.

I don't need to keep count of seizure. I remember the name of numbers whose name is "same."

vs.

We are late to our first stop on our Spring Break Witch Doctor 2019 Tour of Bogotá: Sergio's office. Late because on plane ride down to Bogotá, while boy sleeps, for first time, boy seizes big. Makes noise. Sits up. Arms nailed into wooden corners of ninety degrees. So in the morning we let him sleep in.

At Sergio's, boy gravitates toward massive collection of massive crystals. While boy gravitates, Sergio speaks.

Boy has Hamer point, Sergio insists. *Continue with only happy stories. There is more to seizure, no doubt. But you must address emotional imbalance if you want a happy end.*

Health is about frequency. Correct amplitude, correct range of wave. Boy's frequency is off. Have him recite these numbers, sacred healing codes. You can do it with him. He likes numbers you said. Make the codes a game. 218 the sacred code of the brain. 753 the code for epilepsy. Forty-five times each. These numbers are holy frequencies, good waves that correct bad waves. Restore frequencies to right dimension, as in before.

Give boy essences of specific herbs.

But. There is no doubt more to seizures. Go see my doctor. He will perform biomagnetic reading, restore correct balance to body of boy. If there's something foreign inside un-synchronizing things, he will find. Let's call doctor now. His name is Pedro.

Hello, Pedro. Can you see boy. Sergio looks at us. *Does today work. Today at five.*

We laugh. (No brainer!)

Yes, today. Today at five works fine.

vs.

We arrive at Pedro's office. Sergio's doctor Pedro. It is a small rectilinear two-story house of thin brick combined with concrete block, such as those found in many of the old residential *barrios* of Bogotá. Poured terrazzo floors, dotted with small and large chips of different earth-colored granite rock. Cold and quiet sealed within—the unmistakable damp of the old white brick houses found in several of the circumspect blocks of Bogotá. Bogotá where traffic is so ruthless, where rains so recurrent, that to arrive at destination, even to cold quiet damp white brick house, is to enter setting of ethereal calm.

Hello, we have an appointment with Doctor Pedro, Pedro Gómez, I say.

There is no Pedro here, the older woman with grey bun at the dark wood desk says.

No Doctor Gómez.

No, there is a Doctor Carmona. Carmona Gómez.

What is his first name.

Pedro Gustavo, she says.

Couldn't he be Pedro Gómez. Sergio's doctor.

Well, everyone calls him Gustavo, Doctor Gustavo Carmona.

I am silent.

But, yes, Doctor Carmona is Sergio's doctor. So yes, they are probably the same. Let me check.

Boy's first name is there. Written by hand in pencil on paper upon the 5 o'clock slot.

Wait here, the woman with grey bun says. Stands. Turns. Leaves. *The doctor will call you in.*

We sit on dark wooden bench and wait for Doctor Pedro Gómez/Gustavo Carmona/Pedro Gustavo Carmona Gómez to usher us in.

vs.

At Elizabeth's, Eli's, doctor witch at the heart of my Bogotá, story of boy is told again. She touches her hand to her head, as she does when she is receiving. Twirls hand, fingers of hand,

like a lever by her head. Eli knows us. She sees our faces, paused
before her.

Sweet boy, she says. *Those eyes. Boy knows he is loved. Knows
it too much. We need to reduce manifestations of your indulgent love.
But we will work on that later.*

Today, we have other work. There is something inside boy, she says.
*We need to take boy to special doctor. Doctor will find the something
inside. Find and remove. Do not worry. Boy will be fine. But he must see
this doctor. Doctor who specializes in strange bugs, parasites. Also, boy's
liver is heavy. I'll give you liquid to drink that will clear it. Other drops,
too, to keep you calm. Boy feels your stress—you must endeavor to keep
calm.*

Okay. Okay.

Doctor is strange, she says. *You will like him. You like strange
things. There's one thing.*

What.

Special doctor is a vet.

vs.

Interruption—

Visits to doctors are interrupted. Husband and I sit together, halt.
Share coffee munificent coffee as event of   respite.

Do you hear boy at night, we say. *It is something new: cries boy shouts at
night.*

Perhaps the altitude, we say. *Never first days in Bogotá does anyone sleep
right.*

What to believe, we ask. *All of it: for now, believe all the doctors say.*

It must be coming, nearing, we say, *the pierce of sharp*   *lamplight.*

vs.

At Doctor Carmona's house-office, a dark wooden door opens and the doctor, of exact name uncertain, allows us in.

Doctor Carmona is as quiet as his house. As composed as its white rows of thin brick and cubed block. As calm. As unmoved by the compact traffic of the boundless blocks of Bogotá. He is instantly before us, that rare man who does not want more.

We tell him of seizures of boy. Of what we have learned, the little. Of hospital and diagnosis and prognosis. The little. He agrees on the Keppra: do not give boy Keppra: the way that drug affects the brain is a thing still left to be said. Even after all the decades of administered medication. Keppra is a leaden drug, there are others, better, no doubt.

Doctor initiates a biomagnetic scan. Gently clasps boy's ankles, moving, rotating, gyrating his feet. Doctor is quiet, he wiggles boy's ankles, then leaves feet loose. He himself stands still, marks a paper.

What are you doing, we say.

I am asking boy's body questions. Asking body to tell me what it has. Living or dead, or in between, hidden within. The memory of disease sometimes remains. Inserts itself, camouflages into DNA. *Activates pre-dispositions. Carcass of bug can be as bad as live bug.*

On his paper, a printed list of names. I read. Names of bugs, of bacteria, of virus, of parasites, of fungus. One by one doctor checks or crosses out.

Doctor grins.

The places where things like to hide, he says, with grin. *First rib, big toe, vena cava.*

He does not say what things.

Where is vena cava, I say.

There are two. Two large veins that bring blood from body back into heart. Into heart where blood will be infused with oxygen, then sent back.

What likes to hide, I say.

Disease, he says. *Also, the memory of disease. Parasites, virus, bacteria, cloaked as* DNA.

How do you find it.

I connect with boy. I, in my mind, connect with body of boy, doctor says. *I ask body where the bad stuff lies. I am told what the bad stuff is. I use magnets to move it out of hiding and back into the active blood stream. This is what biomagnetism does. Move disease with magnets to where body can remove.*

What does boy have, I say.

He has prions, which are bad proteins. Parasites and dead parasite shells. Leptospira, a bacteria—this in his liver. Staph. Epstein-Barr. And a fungus, trichophyton, the one that causes athlete's foot.

Is this causing seizures.

I cannot say. It could if it all combines to inflame nerves, other cells in brain. Gliosis is inflammation. MRI *shows what may be gliosis. Inflammation of brain tissue can lead to seizures. The memory of disease, the presence of disease, of infection, of infestation, it can all affect body's electrical currents, its polarity, aggravate the body, its tissues. It is not one thing, but a combination of things that makes people sick.*

I read that same phrase in the Medical Medium, I say.

Which phrase.

It is not the thing, but the combination of.

Then you also read that stress is what is worst of all for body. Emotional and mental stress. For boy to be well, family must be well. For family to be well, family must have faith. Have faith boy will be well and boy will be well.

Yes. Can you treat boy.

I can help, he says. *But, remember, in treatment as in disease, it is not the thing, but the combination of.*

Well, we are definitely doing the combination of, Nelson David says. *Do we need to come back. What's next.*

Yes, come back. I have a machine that does what I am now doing with magnets by hand. Make an appointment with the front desk. I will write the frequencies for machine out for you. Just hand woman at front desk the paper with the frequencies tomorrow, and they will set up machine.

How many times do we need to do it, I say.

I don't recommend more than once per month. After each session, I must reevaluate boy. Check if correctional frequencies have changed. It takes time for body to readjust. Do one now and whenever next you are back in Bogotá, we can do another. One thing.

What, we say.

For thirty minutes boy must lie still. No TV, no cell phones in room. Nothing with electromagnetic field allowed within for it will lessen effect of machine.

This, Doctor Carmona says while boy, sensing he is now free, leaps off examining bed.

Nelson David and I fall silent.

I will work on story, I say. *Will prepare only happy story for boy that day.*

vs.

Incidentally, boy wears same Juventus jersey he wore in the French-doctor emergency room to his first biomagnetic scan.

vs.

Who names the lesser parts of body. Is it first come, first name.

Vena cava is simple. A lazy name, verbatim application of Latin. Hollow vein. Cava as in cave. Vena as in vein. Hollow cave of vein. Where disease hides. The raider's den.

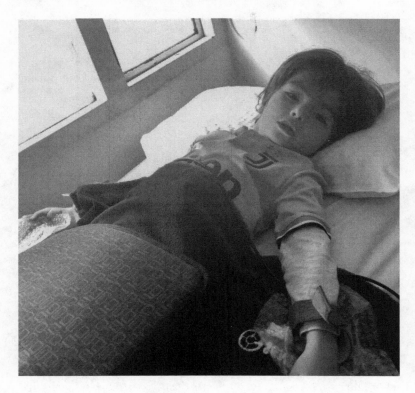

Literal spot where blood, darkened by the body's oxygen consumption, depleted, flows in. Where expense of body connects to replenish of heart. Heart as literal spot of restock, of delivery, of supply for ceaseless demand. Where life is modest, simple as pulley: air pulled down tube by pump of lung. Air drawn in via open cavity of nose, triangle orifice in center of face, permeable slit of skin built-in to render spent blood red.

Disease hiding in literal spot, vena cava, where blood arrives tired after laborious shift. Cells vulnerable, expended. How does disease know where to go. Is it evil or survival. Is there a difference. If so, what.

I believe in God. I acknowledge this to mean I believe there is room enough for all.

vs.

I do not go with husband to office of vet the first time boy visits. I have work to do in Bogotá. Sale of company progresses. There are new spreadsheets to prepare: new boxes with numbers, with figures, to aggregate. To chain. What I work to sell is this: sum as quantity, as congregation, as vendible combination of.

vs.

Husband takes boy to doctor who is vet, the Vet. A doctor not of children but of assorted household pets.

I sit with husband, drink coffee, and husband narrates before he forgets—

It is difficult to understand Vet when he speaks, but not because he is doctor. It is tricky to understand all doctors when they speak. But with Vet, it is harder. He mumbles.

Within Vet's office within his house are statuettes of the Virgin Mary, an entire set of shelves supports them, figurines of religious figures: Pope, Saints, a thick-laid Bible.

Husband tells Vet what is going on. Repeats the story. But now adds mention of the strep, the staph, the Epstein-Barr.

Eli is right, Vet says, *in sending you here. What boy has may be simpler than you fear. Let's see if we can fix this. But I believe Eli is right. Meanwhile give the boy a purgative. I will prescribe three adult doses. It will be strong. But it will flush out whatever it is boy has.*

Vet talks to boy and, somehow, in the talking to boy, draws

blood from boy, from finger of boy, boy who has bitten nail of each finger down to its flesh core. Is it soccer that he talks to boy about. Or is it poster of silly mad scientist dog that hangs from Vet's wall. Husband does not remember. Husband does not even notice blood is drawn until Vet takes vial to a private office behind patient office, which must be, purportedly, Vet's lab.

While you begin purgative, I will draw a culture of bugs within boy's blood, Vet says. *Find the culprit and the density of it.*

Okay, husband say. *When do we call back.*

Come back later this week. I'd like to see him again this week. Come back Saturday morning. Culture will be ready by then.

Okay. Any idea of what boy has.

Do you believe in God, Vet says.

Yes, of course, husband says. *But we are not Catholic in that way.*

While you wait, you must have faith. Have faith and pray. On Saturday we will see what it is boy has.

vs.

Repeat the story. Es. Te. O. Ar. Why.

vs.

I have a friend whose son has something similar to autism. I see her running sometimes. When she runs, she always runs with phone. Clutch grab clasp of phone. I used to sink when I saw this. Because I knew why phone always by her side.

Now my phone always by my side. I don't run. But if I ran, I would run with phone. Clutch grab clasp. Is it distressing to see this grasp of phone happen to us. Is presence of phone sad. Is it.

Certainly, it is new. But phone by side does not hurt. Does

not weigh. It just is. A rectangular entity that dials or rings. There is a why, certainly. A cheerless why, I suppose. Boy is sick. Boy at risk. Sick is sad. Risk is fear. But right now, boy is fine. Seizure apart, phone by side, boy is fine.

What has actually shifted thus far.

There is an ease of slipping into murk, into fear. Magnetic pull of slip. Of down. Gravity of gloom. Wallow as lure. The feeling is there, the fear, the temptation of despair. But the narrative, the chronicle of feeling comes from mind. Mind interprets feeling of sink, crafts a pigment of it through words. Mind can rationalize so as to skirt, engage rise, pursue mount. Boy is fine so long as mother so long as father can maintain climb.

vs.

I approach the word "*prion.*" Carmona's word "*prion.*" Reread notes of what he said. Reread every word every doctor said. Reread to comprehend. Reading comprehension: make sure each word is a word I know well enough to replace with another word. *Prion.* Boy's biomagnetism scan reads "*prion.*" I do not comprehend.

This is what the Centers for Disease Control and Prevention says about prions—

"Prion diseases or transmissible spongiform encephalopathies (TSEs) are a family of rare progressive neurodegenerative disorders that affect both humans and animals. They are distinguished by long incubation periods, characteristic spongiform changes associated with neuronal loss, and a failure to induce inflammatory response.

"The causative agents of TSEs are believed to be prions. The term "prions" refers to abnormal, pathogenic agents that are transmissible and are able to induce abnormal folding of specific normal cellular proteins called prion proteins that are found most abundantly in the brain. The functions of these normal prion proteins are still not completely understood. The abnormal folding of the prion proteins leads to brain damage and the characteristic signs and symptoms of the disease. Prion diseases are usually rapidly progressive and always fatal."

This of course represents little to me other than cause for alarm. Upon reading further, I find that mad cow disease is produced by prions gone mad. Mad cow disease signifies death. I read further still, visit other, more hand-drawn, watered-down sites.

I find that prions are protein particles. Particles because they are not cells—they have no nucleus, no nucleoid, which in cellular language is the same as saying no source of reproduction, of origin, of cradle. They don't even have a means of death. A remnant of life that somehow is indestructible, somehow able to reproduce. Something that isn't quite living, isn't quite dead, but can cause a living brain to malform to death.

Prions are of the body. Protein particles on surface of cells of brain. Prions are not foreign to body, like virus. Yet, something makes prions go rogue. What's more, prions cannot be destroyed, not after years of formaldehyde, of acid, of burn.

vs.

Why is it I am writing these words into book.

vs.

Finally, last on our list of doctors: Elsa, head witch of the mountain-top plateau sprawl of Bogotá. Elsa's office, too, is her home. One-hour-drive up into the cold cloud air beyond the traffic veil of *La Capital*.

Polarity of brain is inverted, she says, *placing magnets by boy's right frontal lobe, right front bend of head. Plus is where minus should be, she says, minus where plus should be.*

I can correct it, she says, but it will not last. Magnets are stubborn. They are difficult to correct in a way that lasts. Did you get the heavy metal tests back.

No, not yet, I say. *Soon.*

It's possible he will have mercury, like you. I remember it was just after his birth that I treated you for it, for that pain that would not go away in your gut.

Mercury gets passed from mother to son, I say. I do not ask: it is fact recently read.

They are many the things we pass to our firstborn child, Elsa says.

What else could he have.

Epstein–Barr is a virus that is strong. That with poor diet, combined, a trigger, perhaps. This is a process: we've only just begun. The polarity in his brain will need to be fixed, permanently affixed. For this, I insist, the Cuban doctor in Guayaquil. The Cuban doctor will come here, to Bogotá, in a month. He will perform scans for patients of mine. Here at my home. Think about it. But don't think too long. The appointments fill up. Meanwhile, no sugar, no dairy, no wheat. Nothing at all that comes from the sea.

What vitamins, I ask. *We are giving so many.* I pull out all the vitamins from my bag.

Let's ask.

One by one, she places each vitamin container in left hand of boy who is lying down. Tells boy to lift right arm while his left hand holds vitamins flat, resting upon cot. She places one of her hands on boy's head, the other presses boy's upheld right arm.

First, Vitamin B complex, chewable berry flavor. Boy holds in left hand. Elsa presses right hand of boy down. Arm stays firm.

Vitamin B is good, she says.

Next, Magnesium, animal shaped, berry flavored as well. Boy holds in hand. Elsa presses down. Arm stays up.

Okay. Magnesium is good.

Next, a kid's brain combo vitamin pack, selenium, zinc, manganese, chromium, animal shaped, citric in flavor. Boy holds in hand. Elsa presses down. Arm stays up.

This one is good, too. Keep it.

Next, a homeopathic German epilepsy formula. Reckeweg R33. The dropper in boy's hand. Elsa presses. Arm drops down.

This is useless. Throw it away.

Finally, belladonna, in homeopathic dispensation as well. Boy's arm stays.

Elsa is surprised. She asks from where, whom, did belladonna come.

Elizabeth, I say.

Elsa nods in recognition, avowal. Belladonna, like perpendicularly extended arm of boy, for now, will stay.

She places magnets, circular disks, on boy's body. Leaves them be. Talks to us, but brief.

Cuban doctor, Russian machine, littoral city of Guayaquil. No one else with this Russian magnet electric body frequency fixing machine. Go to Guayaquil, do not worry. Guayaquil is big, pleasant, fine. Boy will be good. You will be fine. What boy has is electric.

Elsa removes her magnets from boy's brain and shows us polarity. Where before was plus now is minus. Where before was minus now is plus. Polarity of boy's brain corrected.

Re-inverted. Unremarkable, again. Mother and father by boy are silent. But, Elsa hears what mother and father dare not say.

No. It will not stay. The polarity of brain of boy will not keep right. It will go back to wrong. I cannot make it stick. Cuban doctor is coming here to visit Bogotá. In a month, here, in Bogotá. Come back. The doctor will bring a small machine with which to do a scan, a different scan. Meet him. Have doctor give boy this different scan.

I sense it coming, the hounded onset of fine. Of good coffee in cryptic coastal Ecuadorian city of greetings, here we are, and we are fine.

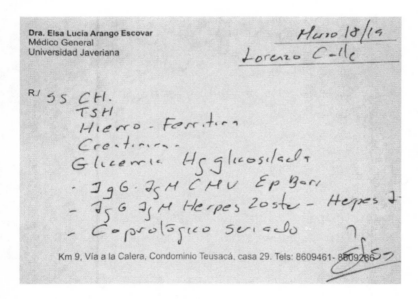

vs.

Tráemelo, again, in one month.

vs.

Thought is of the brain. Emotion is of the heart. Sense is of the brain and heart combined. Logos. Pathos. Ethos. (Nothing new to see here!) I believe I agree with the substance of these words, derived from electric connections formed within brain's folds.[3]

Sentiments and humors are emotions, but subtler. "Humor" comes from Old French, which in turn comes from Latin, *humere*. *Humere* as in moisture, humidity, vapor, subterranean stream. Cloud of sentiment floating, rising to seize mental state of within. State of senti/mentality. Implicit within word is idea that emotions are alien to body. Somehow capable of seizing the body, seizing the brain. Sentiment, humor, emotion: feeling gone rogue, seizing the organ of mind, seizing our expeditor of soul.

Whence before sentiment could not, would not be deliberately named, purposefully owned, today as a culture, we claim. History of melancholy vs. history of sadness is history of what it means to name. Am I wrong to think our naming of feeling has improved. In retrospect, I feel, I am usually wrong.

Thought vs. emotion vs. sense. Feeling vs. sentiment. Melancholy vs. mind.

Premonition. Premonition, though, is different. Portent, foreboding, knowingness. I am certain omen comes from all: omen is of brain, is of heart, is of body, all of it, all of the soul's devices, forcibly combined.

---

3   Again: that I—
             this I—
who is here   who is there
to agree with me or   not;
again: that me—
            this me—
who seeks with words   to explain
what I/I
believe or   do not.

Subterranean embodied stream. Premonition is a lucidity that emerges from the crux, the cross, of it all.

Deus ex machina et al.

vs.

It's remarkable to think that someone sat down and wrote the Bible. It is remarkable. Remarkable to think.

The New Testament and the Old. The Old which contains the Hebrew Torah, also named the Pentateuch, the Five Books of Moses. Because I was raised with Bible as only holy book, I speak only of this one, this single book out of many other holy books.

Even more remarkable to think: several ones sat down to write the Bible, Torah, Old, New Testament, Books of Moses, et al. That we read this book, these many smaller books, as single book: that we read this conglomerate amalgam book with veneration as if it was written by single body, by singular God, when it was written by several hands. Several as they are, the hands of history's arms.

It is this perhaps that is most remarkable. The thought, sentiment, sense, belief that the Bible is, in retrospect and in present, a holy book: assiduously grasped as word of God. The Word of God. Transcribed by human hands, despite.

Belief happens because enough ones over enough years believe: because the many ones said that the Bible was written by God. Belief is part of God and part of people. Self-fulfilling prophecies are part of this: the earthly realm of humankind. Certainly, if there is belief in God, then why not belief in book of God. Weekly pilgrimage, masses who amass to hear printed word of God read by ordained tongue.

It feels good to read with veneration. Good to imagine all the millions of ones over thousands of years who, too, read in veneration. I read in veneration. I am one with the many. With the churches, the temples, the steeples: all the adoration. One with the marble wood mosaic altars upon which lie consecrated copies of hard bound holy books of God.

Congregations who come to abide by words aligned as printed lines. Anything that makes the one feel like the many— like we all are in this together—is typically good. Like the subway when it is silent.

Don Quixote, too, is essentially a collection of aphorisms, but presented as humor rather than as ultimate understanding of ultimate reality (AKA God!). Aphorisms that accompany a story of an old man convinced he is what he is not. It is funny to see him act like what he is not, to encourage him, as readers, to support Don Quixote's false beliefs, because it matters not that he acts like what he is not, it only matters that he believe, that he act, and that, as readers, we are permitted to *ad infinitum* watch.

With *Quixote* we read the story of the belief of one man, upon this belief he commits wild and crazy acts. It is funny, so silly, to see someone believe what he is not—so we watch. With Jesus, it is we who believe, we who read into, we who act upon belief. This act, our act, of belief is to watch, to read, to absorb, to contemplate Jesus' every step, his walk, as an act of God. It is fun, too, I believe, to believe a holy act. But we do not call it fun. We call it faith. Faith is when we believe events are an act of God.

Because no one says that *Don Quixote* is written by the hand of God no one reads this book believing it is the word of God.

But I regard *Don Quixote* in veneration because of the millions of ones over hundreds of years who, too, read and laughed.

Reading and believing vs. reading and laughing probably supply the same amount of wellness on a molecular basis to the one who is reading. Solace cupped as if a book of psalms by the palms of your hands.

vs.

Nothing on internet about Cuban doctor with Russian Cold War magnetic machine capable of redrafting electrical brain in florid heat of Guayaquil.

No proper site with a "Home" and/or a "Contact Us." Nothing, nowhere, like an "FAQ."

What I find: an old press release buried within Presidency of Colombia's official site announcing that a former President gave Cuban doctor Colombian nationality because Cuban doctor cured this President's nephew of seizure disorder.

Elsa insists on Cuban doctor. *It's what I would do*, she says, *if boy was my son.*

Cuban doctor, Russian machine, torrid heat of Guayaquil. Colombian, we discover, not by birth but by decree.

vs.

In Lispector I read about the unsettling nature of happiness. I wonder if this is what Jonathan reads when he thinks of me. Thinks of me so as to incite me to read the book he reads. I wonder because this line prompts me to think of him thinking of me. Of him needing me to read the book he reads.

vs.

Elsa who on first call says what boy has is *le petit mal*. Look it up. *Petit*. Because out there is a *mal* that is *grand*. *Petit* vs. *grand*. They are relative, the terms of *mal*.

vs.

Boy's heavy metal exams, tested from stalks of hair cut close to his scalp, are back from lab. Metals in exam are listed in order of those that cause most to least harm. Levels of metal in boy's hair, consequently, in boy's blood, are not dire.

It is not mercury, Elsa and I say. Say with dismay: mercury not good, but mercury is *mal* that Elsa and diet can cure.

Mercury, in boy's case, not passed from mother to first-born child, though mercury poisoning is a *mal* I had. Too much fish during pregnancy, too much shrimp. Mercury in oceans eaten by fish deposited into my inadvertent bloodstream. Bloodstream that fed boy while boy was fetus, fish within my placental sea.

Mercury poisoning resulted in furtive pain in my gut no doctor, no abdominal scan, could explain. Elsa named upon my first step into her office-home of Bogotá.

Hi, she said. *You have mercury,* she said. *Cut stalks of hair close to scalp, send it to this lab. Meanwhile, purchase chlorella tablets. Spirulina powder, but mix it well, it tastes awfully bad. Nothing from the sea, no sugar, no dairy, no wheat.*

When my labs returned, my mercury levels read ninety-seven percent. I had mercury poisoning, just as Elsa said. An entire year popping chlorella, spirulina. Vegan diet to cull mercury out. Eighteen months later new test of hair cut from scalp came back neat.

Mercury retrograde within my material skin.

vs.

According to *Medical Medium,* no such thing exists as autoimmune disease. What exists inside, within, is external. External virus, external bacteria, external fungus, external parasite, external toxin, such as heavy metal. These things combine with each other, but, more so, with stress. External stress, internalized.

They are rigorous, the vermin of decay: they camouflage, they adapt. They wait for time, exact, attack. They wait within skin, within cell, within molecular worm of cellular DNA.

The body is not dumb. Dumb is not the body. On a cellular level, molecular, and beyond, it knows—senses, presages—infection. Knows of patient invaders, of dormant enemy imbedded in rungs of double helix, the crux of person body embodies.

To attack infection, body attacks itself. Identifies membranes breached, so as to wittingly, in turn, breach. Body is rigorous, too. Onset of unwell emerges. Unhappy host endeavors to return to good, to fine, to day-to-day physical, material well.

A few of many diseases, conditions, called autoimmune—

- Multiple Sclerosis
- Guillain-Barre Syndrome
- Hashimoto's Disease
- Lupus
- Rheumatoid Arthritis

Dumb is not body. Unhappy as host, it endeavors. Despite having to cross boundary, cellular membrane, of what it means to self-inflict. It must get worse to get better. The greater evil is hidden, blended within. Body understands sacrifice. Willingness to dig, knowingness of where. Virus, bacteria, parasite, fungus, heavy metal. Unhappy host endeavors to be well. To hound homeostasis, balance the apparatus of soul.

Body is not dumb. What swells is only the advance, the bruised ranks of withstand, the calculus of specific harm, permeable skin that cedes so as not to succumb.

vs.

From the surgery meant to drain his brain, my father emerges as a new person for us, for me, for himself to meet. Body is same. Name is same. Face is same. But brain is not, so person is not. When his brain is drained of excess blood, part of his self is drained as well.

At times, we thought it was him again sitting in a large chair, ready to read, listen to Schubert, smoke a pipe, sneak a drink. Father come back, come back to tell us all. But then we tried talk and talk did not work.

Quién, he says when he hears us talk, hears us speak. *Qué. Cómo.* He says, often, softly.

Does not expect answers to the words of question, sometimes the only words he sounds.

Who. What. How. This is what father wants to know.

Who father is, what father is, how. Who father is now, and what. What happened and how.

When is not a question because when has an answer. When. Never. Never forever again.

vs.

An onset of thought emerges within skin, within mind, both material, both mine—

> I will not miss seizure of boy when gone
> But I will miss writing of book when done

Because of this thought I confirm my routine faith. I operate predictably as a day-to-day person of faith. Seizures of boy will be gone. Writing of book will be done. Faith is not versus. It is sovereign. I believe in God. Oh, so private, so prosaic, this chronic faith of mine.

vs.

Incidentally,
I occur   at the exact,   literal,
                    intersection of J. Alfred   Prufrock
                    and   Colombia,
the country specifically spelled
                                          as such.

vs.

In Colombia, weekends with a Monday off are called *puentes*. *Puente* means "bridge." As in, colloquially, hey, going any-where for *puente*. For *puente*, I stay. Or, go here. Go there.

    We—Nelson David, boy, I—are here. Here. In Bogotá. On a Saturday *puente* morning, here, in Bogotá. *Puente* week-ends are the best time to navigate Bogotá, the only time. The city empties down into warmer mountains east west north south. Bogotá is set nine thousand feet up inside the sky. It is wintry up so high in the Andes: cold, rainy, enduringly damp. Drive down from Bogotá's plateau for two hours and already it is lush, opulent, elatedly warm. The air smells of secret animal life. Colors dart: the breasts of little birds, wings of butterflies, backs of poison frogs. Pogo stick hops of absurd insects. Excess heaves beneath the shade of banana trees hung like the groins of ancient fertility gods.

Meanwhile, Bogotá empties. Empty Bogotá is glorious Bogotá. Grid-free. Gray-free. We flow easy early to good coffee place. Venezuelan-owned. More and more Bogotá is Venezuelan-owned. Venezuelan good coffee place reminds us of Lucy.

Lucy with whom we recently spoke, who says Venezuela now, even during bright days is dark as done. Lucy who called to ask about boy despite her dark. *Something with boy's small intestine*, she says. *Tell me, how does boy evacuate.*

Barely, we say. *Just barely.*

His intestine is dry. Give boy mineral oil. He needs to eliminate. Irrigate intestine to help him empty whatever may be inside.

In Venezuelan-owned good coffee place. Sunny Saturday *puente* morning in Bogotá. We remember what our Lucy from done Venezuela phones to say. We need to remember so much so many have said.

We pay. Get up to go. Mineral oil on hold. For now, it is time for us to see the Vet.

vs.

The vestibule of Vet doctor's office-house is a corridor perpendicular to street, with a bench upon which people and their pets sit. One side of corridor is open to interior patio with grass and path. The path leads to altar of Virgin Mary, who holds baby Christ with one arm. Virgin Mary wields, draws, pools us, in.

We look at her, us three, walk the short path to her. We summon a short prayer in Spanish that we know by heart how to recite by mouth. We cross ourselves. We linger. Dawdle. We have nothing left to say but we stay.

The Church probably ruined Mary for me. Tarnished her with virginity as brandish, as sacrosanct. I think to tell boy story of Mary, why life was so hard for her: the story of a mother with a special son. Why special is difficult. But I don't. I do not. I am quiet. Then silent. We all are silent. I sense—perhaps we all do—the boundary, the aura between quiet and silence. It is a margin, a basin, a vessel that is full.

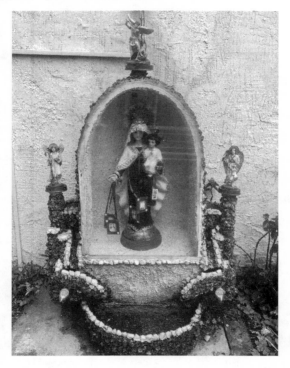

vs.

Of all the manifestations of the Virgin Mary, the one I am most familiar with, the one I am able to recognize pointblank if I encounter on sidewalk, is Virgin of Guadalupe. *La Virgen de Guadalupe.* This despite the fact that Virgin of Guadalupe is of Mexican origin, and there is a Colombian manifestation of the Virgin Mary, also based on an apparition.

La Virgen de Chiquinquira serves the upper pleats of the Andes range and is named after a small town a few hours north by snaking mountain road from the traffic block grid of Bogotá.

Still, I wouldn't know the difference between her and, say, the Virgin of Lourdes on a street corner.

vs.

Quiet dark office of Vet seems real in the exact opposite way masses of people, crowded events, do not. Here is life laid carefully on the shelf. Life with purpose put forth.

Boy has tough parasite, Vet says, hands us paper with name. *He has it in concentrated amount.*

Can it be removed.

Yes of course. You are removing it already with the purgative I gave you. The Albendazole.

Yes. We gave him the drug.

After you purge, you must give him some drops. New ones I will prepare. Erase memory of parasite from cells.

Okay.

Then go to Elizabeth, she will restore until well. The rest is in her hands.

She reorganizes his cells, I say.

You can see it that way. Or this. Vet gets up and takes down thick leather Bible from his Saint and Virgin Mary shelf.

He opens Bible to Ecclesiastes Chapter 38 and bids I read, starting from verse nine—

9. "My child, when you feel ill, don't ignore it. Pray to the Lord, and he will make you well.

10. Confess all your sins and determine that in the future you will live a righteous life.

11. Offer incense and a grain offering, as fine as you can afford.
12. Then call the doctor—for the Lord created him—and keep him at your side; you need him.
13. There are times when you have to depend on his skill.
14. The doctor's prayer is that the Lord will make him able to ease his patients' pain and make them well again."

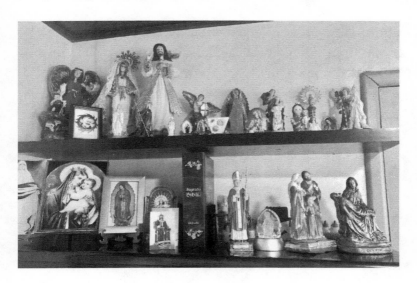

You said you have faith, Vet says when I finish.
    Yes.
    Then pray. Have faith. If not, boy will sense your stress.
    What about Keppra, I say.
    What about it.
    Do we give boy Keppra.
    What for.
    We continue to see six to ten seizures a day.
    Finish the purgatives. Give boy drops. He should recover. Have faith. Pray to God.

We leave—we are not sure what to believe. We are hopeful of course. And then there are all the books, all the words I've recently read. All we've asked; all doctors have said. It could be, it could: that build-up of toxins affected electrical pathways of brain.

Getting into car I say to husband, *Western medicine needs to reconnect with God. I think at a moment in history it needed to disconnect, in order to advance. But now it needs to reconnect. In order to advance.*

Vet said those same words the first time I went, husband says.

You didn't mention it.

I forgot. But he said, basically, what you just said. That Western medicine had lost its link to God. That it needed to recover its connection to God.

I am quiet. Then say, *what do you think of doctor. Of what doctor said.*

I do not doubt boy has parasite. I do not doubt it is good to remove parasite. I don't know if that will remove the seizures though. We will have to see.

I am quiet.

Doctor is a scientist, husband says. *Empirical despite the religiosity. Let's see.*

5

Mommy, It Hurts: A Five-Paragraph Essay on Maternal Fault[4]

I, like my son, am no better than myself (Ana María Caballero)

In this essay, I will attempt to demonstrate that seizures of boy are entirely my fault. Here, I refer to both fault of, I, the mother and, I, the Mother.[5] Boy's seizures are my fault, as well as the fault of system of Mother. I do not explore the role of predisposition—of genetic, structural, congenital or otherwise built-in

---

4   Maternal fault, as approached here, is not to be confounded with maternal guilt. Fault, as approached here, is to be understood as acceptance of fact. As finger pointed, but not crooked, hob-knuckled finger. I accept that illness of boy might be a direct result of choices I made while raising boy. I made wrong choices. It is my fault. I move, stand, advance to correct wrong choices. Procedure of reverse. Writing of self-adjust.

5   Failure of System of Mother is intended to be understood as failure of system that principally charges one parent, from within the union of two parents, with care of young children, regardless of gender. System of Mother refers to the still socially prevalent archetype of the figure of the mother as giver, as lone adult responsible for the proper raising of a couple's brood. Even if lone adult works or wants to write, lone adult is implicitly liable for the well-being of children that are equally the responsibility of another adult who somehow is less accountable for proper nutrition, healthy activities, day-to-day medical care of child. I do not attempt to enter here into the problematics of the existence of such System. There will be other books for that.

flaw—that may lie within the skin-frame of boy. Predisposition is not included in this discussion of maternal fault, not even predispositions of the congenital kind, which inherently derive from Mother, from me, as biological parent, because this exploration posits that predisposition alone is not sufficient to launch seizure. Environmental triggers are necessary in order to bring forth onset of epilepsy of boy. Triggers can be translated as lack of nurture, which results in nature, built-in, rousing, convulsing, awake. In the three years prior to seizures of boy, I was employed in the salvaging of a family company dedicated to the importation and distribution of wine into the country specifically spelled as Colombia. The salvaging of company, while I was living outside of Colombia, was very difficult. As a result, I could not properly care for boy. I resorted to any electronic device that appealed to boy, any type of food solicited by boy, including and especially sugar, as it was the most violently in demand, the most likely to be received by and consumed in silence, accepted any antibiotic offered by doctors for any ailment of boy big or small anything to get boy back to school so I could focus on work. For three years, at least, I nurtured, electronically, dietarily and medically onset of seizures of boy.

Electronic devices emit electromagnetic frequencies that affect the innate electromagnetic fields of body. Body is designed to withstand electromagnetic interference when body is in healthy state. However, an excess of electromagnetic devices can negatively affect a physically compromised body. Additionally, electronic hand-held devices, such as iPads, such video games, such as YouTube's short-duration videos generate visual stimulation that can potentially instigate seizures. Although a predisposition must be there, the visual stimulus can result in release of built-up electrical energy in brain via seizure. Because mother is busy, Mother is absent. Because Mother is absent no one in home bothers to read about electromagnetism. Electromagnetism of body is real. Real phenomenon. Electric body, a closed circuit of energy that flows when positive and negatively charged electrons move each other around so as to grow, move, think, sleep, work. Magnetism of body is invisible by definition. This is not to defend the mother giving the child the iPad so consistently so. Who if not her, her of witch doctor faith, should apprehend that metal object in hand powered by electricity hour after hour, day after day, morning after morning, evening after evening afternoon after afternoon, would eventually cause decay. Who if not her, her, the witch doctor mother, should suspect that energy of body flows down up around down and that apparatus in hand, foreign as such, would eventually invert flow. Who if not her. Only her. I, the mother and Mother, knew the bill would come. But I knowingly gave child phone, television, iPad, Nintendo, whatever to occupy child so I could save company and just give me one more week. One more dozen afternoons. Boy consumed. In his hands, a piece of metal lit up. His body, flawed or not, acquired the parameters of metal, in his hands, lit up. The grid of flow of energy of his young boy body overlapped with the grid of flow of energy of electric object, day in day out. Polarities capsized. Biological charge and material discharge. Invisible all of it. Meanwhile momma, the witch doctor momma, she, I, we sensed, oh, we knew. Bought silence.

Sugar, processed sugar, feeds viruses, bacteria, fungi, parasites in the human body. It numbs the immune system, weakening its ability to focus on what's at stake. When a body wants sugar, it is the bad stuff in the body asking to live, to survive. Virus, remarkable, somehow becomes thought. Becomes beg. Becomes want. Becomes physical request, cry, hand of boy stretched out asking mommy mommy, mimi, mama, mami, give me cookie. Give me candy. Give me cake. Organism subjugated to stamina of disease. Family unit orbiting the gravity of disease. Child, cookie jar, mother, a solar system of future physical ail. Mother dispensing sugar as appeasement of want, child's want of Mother, of mother's time, Mother's time that is not the mother's because of mother's excessive work. You want mommy, here, have a chocolate cookie in the meantime, little boy. Ice cream after school, before dinner, post doctor. 7-Eleven Warhead full bag to dispense over one or two days. Candy is part of young. Sugar part of grow. Culturally it is everywhere. Every holiday. Part of the curriculum. Part of each good coffee place. Boy asks for sugar: Mother gives, we give. Here, boy, eat, now please let mommy finish her work in peace.

If boy gets sick, boy cannot go to school or engage in after-school. Ill boy at home requires constant attention. Trip to doctor, to drugstore, to market. At least once. To each one. Monitoring of fever. Of food. Of pee and poop. Sleep declines or adjourns. During day boy wants only mother. Even if boy entertained, during fever lull, boy wants me. By boy's side only the Mother. Mother by ill boy cannot work. I cannot work. Cannot save company. Sick boy despite, there is company. At first sign of fever past one hundred degrees, I make appointment at pediatrician. If antibiotics are offered as option, they are accepted as requisite. Keep boy well so boy can return to school so mother can work on saving Mother's company. Antibiotics, which kill all: bad bacteria and good: the good bacteria that helps ward future disease. We will deal with the future in the future, mother says. When the company is saved. Presently, deal to sell the company is being brokered. Company for sale because Mother saved. Boy's future, too, is present: I deal with the present. With him, I continue toil of save.

I have shown in this essay how seizures of boy are my fault. Fault of mother. Fault of caretaker, fault of protector, and, as such, fault of System of Mother. Too busy mother is Failure of System of Mother. Seizures resulted as a result of poor diet, over-indulgence of electronic devices and exploitation of antibiotics. Regardless of potential underlying propensity of convulsion within physical material framework of body of boy. Boy developed seizures during trough of bad diet, electronic apparatus abuse and misapplication of antibiotics. Indeed, boy had recently taken antibiotics, days before onset of seizures. Boy was eating little real food during day at school and sugar-packed snacks in afternoon. Other than breakfast and dinner no substantive nutrition entering blood of boy. Antibiotics however entering blood of boy. Electronic device lit up held by hand of boy. Mother considered some fallout would come, but later, lighter. By then she would be good mother. Perhaps have time to dissuade future, become present. But boy's body weakened and became unable to self-regulate. Unable to keep electronic impulses in balance. Unable to daunt disease. Weakness made manifest. Seizure as ultimate warning for mother and Mother to heed. Take better care of boy. Take actual care of boy, seizures say. Accept fault so you, so Mother, so I, can look after boy: employ functional affection, actuate protection, obtain remedy, foster, encourage, nurture boy as if it were my only job.

6

In terms of telling of story, eventually anything continual, disruptive or not, gets old. Story gets old. New becomes norm. Norm becomes dull. Dull as in perpetual chagrin. Dull, even, this recurrent, repetitive shiver of boy.

Even vastly great things manage to get so overused, so over-worn, they become done. Greatness wears off, gets tired, retires. But, so long as you consider the object apart from its myriad manifestations, infinite iterations, consider just the object, just the first incidence of mind behind object's birth—its unmed-iated true form—the object remains great. Grand. Not dull, but pure. Blunt rock uncut: spasm of spring.

Faithfully admiring great things after they get old is an invi-tation to rise above saturation, above reiteration, above the norm of compulsively new. For example: Andy Warhol silver screens (can't tell them apart no more).[6] Or certain lines written by the studious hands of T.S. Eliot. You just can't refer to them anymore because: seriously. Not again. Do something different to do it right. Supporting documentation is valid if not yet cat-alogued, roped as a volume, anthologized.

O, to be a virgin, touched for the very first time. Like an Eliot virgin. He's so fine, and he's mine. Makes me strong, yeah, he makes me bold. I'd been had. I was sad and blue. But he makes me feel. Yeah.

He makes me feel.

---

6 (David Bowie, it was David Bowie who couldn't tell them apart no more.)

&

In terms of progress, I must refer to frequency. On the day I ran to ER with boy, frequency of seizures was eight. As I sit and write, frequency of seizures is four. Inclusive of night. Before we did not know how to count what happened at night. So, eight might actually have been more.

Four today means two during day and two during night. At night boy sleeps with us in little side bed. When seizure hits boy sits up. Talks. Says shouts screams wails a random thing. Then sleeps.

Because of reduction of frequency I can say "progress." Say it and mean it. It is not lie, innocuous lie, used in place of having to say, to respond, to remark: to elaborate.

"Progress" is word I stamp upon envelope of now.

&

In terms of making the best of it, at least boy's seizures are laughter. They are not crying seizures. They are laughing seizures. They are not funny, but they are laughter. I do not consider out loud how laughter of boy has become portent of hazard.[7]

I fasten centrifugal, outwardly twirling thoughts to how seizure of boy is laughter of boy. At least & despite. How unprovoked laughter of boy is better than unprovoked wild flailing of boy on floor with manually inserted substance up the butt because passageway of throat may be shut. All options of seizure placed on scale of measurable quantities of bad. Bad is

---

7   (I only consider deep within how laughter of boy is now sullied laughter: contamination of outward manifestation of joy of boy.)

worse than what we have. What we have is not that bad. Not too bad. Only *petit* bad. We must be grateful for seizures we have.

&

In terms of only happy story, friend whose now two-year-old baby Anaya has cancer, baby whose cancer is in fact stage four neuroblastoma, friend and baby who were in hospital where husband and I, too, were with boy. This friend. This baby. After radiation treatment in New Jersey, receive good news.

Anaya's new scans after radioactive beam directed, focused, somehow inserted, are clear. As in EEG clear. As in Holter monitor clear. As in absence of mass malformed within folds of brain where electrical signal is sovereign. Good news: sparkling, carbonated, animated, remarkable news.

This story parallel to mine, to ours. A tandem of medical clinical days-to-days. Analogous story of unwell child.

Only happy can only be only if this baby well. Anaya well. Boy well. Do I write to command, to affirm, to announce single story of well.

&

In terms of less is more, no one beats DNA. Not one, no single living or inanimate thing. Beats as in surpasses: infinite simple iterations populate bio-diverse, bio-logical life. Four organic molecules: adenine, thymine, cytosine, guanine. Each molecule represented by one letter: ATCG. Adenine goes with thymine; cytosine with guanine. A &. T vs. C & G. Over and over & over again, infinite times. So generous, this combination of:

ATCG
4ever

Inner logic of life: ATCG manifests as all forms of terrestrial, aquatic, aerial existence. All its predispositions. Its sundry conditions.

Four letters to determine your type. Four letters to spell out your story. Here you go: type.

&

In terms of more or less, virus is, more or less, alive. Virus defined as a strand of DNA and/or RNA that needs other, a host, to replicate. Science does not agree if virus is a thing that counts as living. The question is not if virus is dead. The question is if virus is alive. It cannot self-reproduce. It requires host, an alternate version of itself, to reproduce. Not alternate as in male vs. female. Rather, an altogether otherworldly host.

Yet, in terms of definitions, just how different is virus from myself. I, a strand of DNA, with supporting strand of RNA, who, too, cannot self-replicate. To create child, male seed is required. I who swells as host.

&

In terms of what is less, what is more, a jellyfish and a human are on equal living terms. All of us equally alive. On this, no internet forum dispute.

&

In terms of more is more, I must mention Freud. Sum of what I've read is, I am certain, the being within, the monologue, the metaphysicality of who I am. Books read in past serve as backstory to story I presently write, as undercurrent to current, as stream of thoughts of mind.

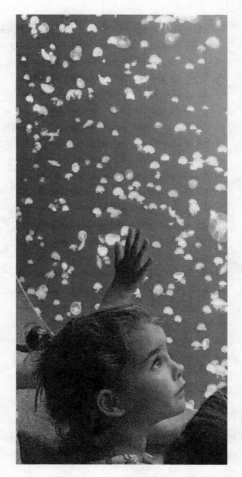

Freud is now embarrassing. It's embarrassing to mention Freud. Seriously: in this day-to-day and day and age. Not Freud, again.[8]

So, I will be brief about Freud, brief as brief about Freud can be. Listicle, here, useful as function of form.

---

8   (Nor Andy Warhol silver screens!)

1. *Unheimlich*: out of place seizure of laughter of boy is *unheimlich*. *Unheimlich*: translates as "uncanny." *Heimlich*, German, means "hidden" and, at the same time, "familiar." Hidden & familiar. *Unheimlich* means "unhidden" and, at once, "unfamiliar." The evident reality of unfamiliar world.

    • "Canny" does not mean "hidden." "Canny" means "clever." "Uncanny" does not mean "unclever." German is better at cleaving, at crafting words that mean horrifying, at defining instant when that which belongs hidden becomes precipitously, chillingly, unhidden. Premonition-like.

    • Sigmund Freud wrote essay on this in 1919, same decade Eliot birthed my beloved Prufrock. His essay is called, "The "Uncanny"" (original double quotes by Freud) and the first sentence is this—

    • "It is only rarely that a psychoanalyst feels impelled to investigate the subject of aesthetics even when aesthetics is understood to mean not merely the theory of beauty, but the theory of the qualities of feeling."

    • Laughter of boy provokes: high-quality feelings of unfunny, uncanny, unknown.

    • Sublimation as Art: lack of sex equals art. Freud composed this statement, this equation.

    • I read Freud's essay on sublimation as required reading for a Master's in Fine Arts writing program at Colombia's largest public university: the National University, *La Nacional*. A sprawling red-brick/green-tree campus in the traffic fog core of Bogotá. There was a lot of Freud in program. A lot of Freud on lack of sex becoming art.

- The class packed with loads of students reading loads of Freud while struggling to create their loads of art. Set to the pulse of the devotedly communist urban grounds of Colombia's *La Nacional*.
- Freud's word for process whereby lack of sex is turned to art is *sublimation*. Sublimate as in absorb so as to reroute. As art. Also: writing, forming, as if possessed. As in, I did not know all this text was within myself: but it was. Art as masturbation. Stroking a physical urge out.
- Instant gratification is theory's conceptual core: if we don't get what we want we turn to art. Many are now gratified in terms of food, shelter, drink. But sex might lack. If not gratified, we turn to thinking about why it is exactly that we are alive. Thinking about meaning is precondition of art. The converse, of course: if we are never hungry and always have access to sex, we will not turn to art. Perhaps this false converse is why Freud is embarrassing now.[9]
- Regardless, Freud's books, his thoughts, are in my head, so when post-hospital-diagnosis-of-epileptic-boy coincides precisely with sudden onset of writing this book, I consider the sublimation of Freud.
- Could it be that absolute lack of sex due to worry derived from uncanny laughter of boy transmutes into text of book, of book flat within your hands, book that would like to thank the author, author's partner, for unreserved lack of fuck.

---

9 Many a successful painter has had access to many a good fuck.

&

In terms of sublimation, I begin to wonder if lack of sugar in children, if absolute confectionary prohibition transmutes, also, into art. Replacing, in Freud's equation, sex with sugar. Both sugar and sex forms of physical, material, short-lived gratification, exaltation, surge.

In other words—

Adult equation: no sex equals hunt for art

Child equation: no sugar equals hunt for sugar in art

Let me explain—boy and Nina Real, both, are likely in candy, sugar, sweat treat physical surge withdrawal. Because shortly after all sugar eliminated from their diets, both become instantly obsessed with *Charlie and the Chocolate Factory*.

First, they adhere to Tim Burton version, the one with Johnny Depp. Then, the Gene Wilder original. When parents tire of Depp, then tire of Wilder, parents find a third. *Tom & Jerry's Willy Wonka*.

Nina Real stops being dog and becomes Willy Wonka. Except she says, Hilly Wonka. Her favorite Wonka is Depp. Wilder somehow is not her Wonka. She requests we put on her cold weather coat and asks for hat, round purple child glasses. Demands we repeatedly play opening scenes of lavish chocolate poured.

Children, mine, no longer ask for candy. They ask for Wonka. We make golden tickets. We tell each other, we scream to each other: *Violet you are turning violet*. We look online for round purple child glasses.

Nina Real learns the Oompa Loompa dance, her favorite, the one that follows Augustus Gloop's fall into Wonka's dark chocolate river.

In the morning, though, she prefers Tom & Jerry to Depp. Depp is for bedtime. Makes sense. Wilder only gets played per request of boy. Boy bonds with gentler shade of Wilder. Nina Real wakes, no longer barks *woof woof*, instead asks for Willy Wonka Kitty Cat. *Hilly Wonka Killy Cat,* she says. Promises to eat banana and oatmeal on plate but please I must play Hilly Wonka Killy Cat.

Banana on plate vs. candy on plate. Sugar vs. sex. Roald Dahl, Freud, what they did was express the obvious: what we forbid finds a way.

&

In terms of ultimate reality, there is chemistry.

Chemical composition of the body, for the most part, is little bits of this: oxygen & carbon & hydrogen & nitrogen & calcium & phosphorus. To a much lesser degree, in the body there are also little bits of: potassium & sulfur & sodium & chlorine & magnesium. Eleven types of elemental atomic atoms combined into the thing. Into combination of.

Other basic elements also present in the body: minerals required by body to do its work. Pinch of zinc. Dash of cobalt. In terms of chemistry, we are same. Things around us, too, uncannily similar in their atomic similarity. For example, the Keppra molecules, sitting so quiet, so patient, atop my cabinet shelf, look like this:[10]

---

10 All molecular graphics taken from the u.s. National Library of Medicine, National Center for Biotechnology Information: https://pubchem.ncbi.nlm.nih.gov

Sucrose, sugar of commerce, looks like this:

Glucose, sugar of body, looks like this:

Lactose, sugar of cow, looks like this:

Vitamin C, harbinger of good, looks like this:

Caffeine (AKA good coffee!) looks like this:

Gluten, so hard for some to digest, looks like this:

Omega-3, so good for boy's brain, looks like this:

A DNA molecule (AKA ultimate you!) looks like this:

Finally, I encounter a satisfying difference: a molecular, granular, particular, quantum other. Table salt, gathered in its shaker, when amplified, elaborated, looks like this:

$Na^+ Cl^-$

&

In terms of ultimate understanding of ultimate reality, there is God. God as thought: God as word. God as human act. Act of faith: individual choice. I choose to enact, to possess faith.

Have faith, my witch doctors say, *pray*. I return to prayer, apply human faith.

&

In terms of ultimate understanding of ultimate reality, there is also quantum physics, quantum mechanics. Science of infinitely small applied to infinitely grand. Science of distance: understood not as spatial, but as dynamic, energetic distance. The distance between atoms, the distance between an electron and its proton, the distance between a planet and its sun, the distance between what you have and what you want. All distance as volition. All vacuums as active.

Astrophysicists explain behavior of vacuum by saying, in fact, space is not empty but filled with dark matter and dark energy. Not dark, as in devoid of light. Rather, invisible. Invisible but detectable. Detectable because it affects what is visible. Galaxies, their planets, their distance vs. each other expands, gravity of heavenly bodies, despite. The universe is growing too fast, instead of collapsing, as we once thought, despite the force of gravity that makes things drop.

Quantum manifestation is not science. It is hokey pokey.

Hokey pokey based on science. Yet: my way into God is this. Atomically, entire known astronomical biological chemical universe is mostly, atomically, the same. Yet: infinite variety. Infinite understandings of infinite realities.

Meanwhile, both atomically and galactically: infinite abundance of empty space. Empty space within atom is proportional to empty space in outer space. Empty space is not empty: it drives galaxies apart. Infinite emptiness wherein microscopic particles coalesce into this or that combination of. Manifestation of.

What if. The strings of heaven, of its bodies, are pulled by hand, by virtue of God. Could it be: God as vacuum: vacuum as God.[11]

Quantum manifestation says this: you can activate the vacuum. Out of infinite possibilities, invoke one. Summon the energy of the vacuum into the outcome you want. Have faith, believe boy will heal. Thought as lamplight flashed into infinite dark: mind as finger that plucks, that tugs, a specific string, an explicit chord, of God.

You do the hokey pokey & you turn yourself around. That's what it's all about.

&

In terms of basic reality, the reality is that sick boy is arduous, exhausting to parent. The surfaces of reality are dented, jagged: it is hard to parent a demanding boy who is at once a seizing boy. Boy is rebel: an anatomy of defy.

When boy sleeps in parents' bed and wakes and shouts and

---

11 (Is synapse of neuron technically a vacuum. I must remember to ask boy's doctors.)

seizes it is hard but also easy. Easy because feelings are clear. Clear-cut emotion of parental desperation.

But, when boy wakes, there are days boy only disobeys. Kicks cousin, kicks sister, kicks mother. Me. Mimi. Kicks me, his mother. Over and over & over. *Boys are boys,* boy's grandmothers, *abuelas,* say. Okay. But, at what point is there a limit crossed. Threshold, aura of problem penetrated.

My dysplasia kids become my ADHD kids, boy's pediatrician has said.

Boy's seizures are not behavioral. They are real, a symptom that is. At school, boy concentrates, sits. But can be physically impulsive, moody, aggressive. I am that mother, the mother who learns not to ask teachers how day went.

It's always better to pull than to shove, the *abuelas* say. *Boy is vigorous, vibrant. Full of life.*

Mother listens. Lets it be. Lets it slide. But I do not want to repeat mistakes of the past. I apply retrospect as foresight to the letting of things slide.[12] I, the mother, stand by: stand guard. Monitor with hope but open to perceive: the point at which boy's behavior becomes another problem that is.

&

In terms of parallel reality, there is Eliot, there is the lamp, the pacifying light of his poems.

&

In terms of terms, the etymology of "epilepsy" is this: two parts, two terms, two words, both Greek, *epi* & *lambanein. Epi* is

---

12 In terms of retrospect, of past reality applied to present, *see Chapter 5.*

everywhere: epidermis, epilogue, epithet, epidemic, epidural, epicenter, epitaph, epistemology, episode, epigenetics. Epi can mean all of these things: over, under, on top of, near, before, after, toward, against, among, upon.

Epi, a term of secondary location in reference to primary location of primary thing. It is not a term of during, of within, of inside. Not even a term of through. It is a term of before and/or after, over and/or under, toward and/or against. It is a term of versus.

Problem is *lambanein* is also secondary in its operation. It means all of these things: to overtake, to seize, to attack, to lay hold of. Lay hold of what. Overtake whom. Attack what.

Lambanein evolved into stem of word, into core: *leps, lepsis*. *Epi+lepsis*. Location in terms of attack. Temporality in terms of take.

If "epilepsy" were sentence, sentence would be without subject, without object. There is only verb, preposition. Action and direction. The act of asking with question, absent. Boy seizes. Boy is over/toward/before/after/near/against-taken. Who is taken. By whom. For whom. The word does not tell what it means.

"Epilepsy," sum of parts, is one definable word whose definition has evolved because it describes a medical clinical disease whose understanding, too, has evolved. "Falling sickness" was the native term in English for the disease before "epilepsy" grabbed hold. Falling sickness is clear in that it does not hide meaning it does not have. You are sick because you fall.

&

In terms of entomology, parasites are not necessarily insects, but some insects rank as parasites. Parasite is simply a living organism that feeds off host: unhappy, the host. Such as flea, tick, or lice. Microscopic parasites subsist inside.

On Saturday morning Bogotá *puente* visit, Vet confirms boy has parasite. In Spanish called *sarcosystina*. Parasite from animals: pig or cow. *Sarcosystina* within boy's skin in focused, resolute amounts. Always not the thing—but the combination, the amassment of. Together with bacteria, with virus, with heavy metal, parasite can disrupt body, nerves, even brain.

Has boy been to farm. Has boy eaten pig. Has boy eaten cow.
Yes. No. What. We don't know.

Vet makes clear: it is never the animal's fault. We who touch, we who eat, we who do not wash hands after we touch and eat.

One thing, for now, is clear: start the purge: remove bug from boy.

&

In terms of terms & conditions, seizure is both.

&

In terms of you & me, the Vet explains statistics well—

If I eat one chicken, and you eat no chicken, statistics will claim that we both ate half.

Half of all epilepsy is idiopathic, its underlying reason, its pretext unknown. If your epilepsy is of cause unknown but mine is of origin known, then both of our epilepsies are each half unknown.

The affliction of one versus vigor of other, statistically, equals infirmity of all. Of the one. Of the other. Of the one that becomes other by virtue of statistical cluster.

&

In terms of odds, Notre-Dame burns down in Paris on same day I pick up first round of boy's DNA results. My immediate attempts to decode text of DNA fail. I stop. Watch Notre-Dame burn.

Inside, invoke help: who in medical, clinical DNA world will shed lamplight on shadow words on DNA page.

&

In terms of coincidence, the day Notre-Dame burns is first day since day I noticed episodes of boy that boy has no episodes. Co-incident-ly. Faith, history, affixed to place, aflame. Possible, always, an episode occurred at school. Boy forgot to recall, remark, admit, avow. Spire of wood, a candle tendered, tethered to sky, ablaze. He usually has one right before sleep. Torrid incandescence of too much lamplight. Not tonight. Asleep at once. Notre-Dame burns. A fire, on fire, afire. Faith aghast, God aglow. Tomorrow, by the light of day, we will know what to proclaim.

&

In terms of uncanny coincidence, episodes of day shift to night on the night Notre-Dame burns. Episodes stronger. Much. Different, too. Boy sits up, shouts in sleep. Sagas of soccer. Russia eliminates Spain in most recent World Cup. *Russia won, Russia won,* sleeping boy screams. *Spain lost, Spain lost,* sleeping boy screams. We call boy by name. He wakes or seems to wake. Does not respond to name. Asks for water. Water is served. Boy drinks: collapses into sleep. Cavernous, silent asleep. Parents wake, hollow, gaping, gasping awake.

I try again, on that sleepless first night-seizure night,

to decipher DNA test. It cannot be chance seizures shift to night on exact day I obtain DNA results. There is one strip of text I am able to read and comprehend:

"Causes Autosomal Dominant Nocturnal Frontal Lobe Epilepsy."

Nocturnal, I get.

Last night, entering bed, I wrote—

"Tomorrow, by the light of day, we will know what to… affirm."

Tomorrow is now today. By the first light of today's day, Notre-Dame has burned. By the first light of today's day, "Nocturnal Epilepsy" is a term I highlight with the hope of grasping what it is I might proclaim.

&

In terms of night & day, night seizures are better than day seizures because of swimming, bicycles, scooters, jungle gyms, soccer practice, play dates, birthday parties, trampolines, anything related to snow and ice, horses, stairs, school, day-to-day walking—especially busy sidewalks—backless chairs, high restaurant stools and other people, particularly those who startle and stare.

Night seizures preclude bunk beds and sleepovers. Curtail hours of sleep for parents of night-seizing-boy. But here the list ends. The list of little things that are better because of night-seizing-boy is longer, so better, than list of little things that are curbed, trimmed, clipped from life of family of night-seizing-boy. It is a measure of business, the business of progress, of forward, of positive growth.

Doctors confirm night seizures not more hazardous than day seizures, so long as boy does not fall from bed. We buy earplugs. Sleep in boy's room. Leave boy in our room, where bed is bigger, and boy during night seizure is free to flail. We, parents, sleep some. The list of little things that are better grows.

For example: Siri. Boy discovers Siri. Asks Siri what Siri thinks over and over hoping to get answers boy wants. For example, who Siri thinks is the world's best soccer player (Messi!), or worst (Ronaldo!).

Boy asks Siri, *Siri do you think that you're a chicken butt*.

I tell boy, *Siri does not think, Siri only knows*.

Siri do you know that you're a chicken butt.

I don't have an answer for that.

Siri is graceful when she does not know. We laugh. Laughter of all, within correct context, correct combination of fun.

&

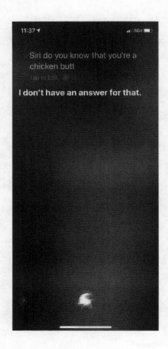

In terms of wrong combination of fun, for Jonathan silence was empty space, dark vacuum to fill up. To occupy: urgently, constantly, with talk, with book, with stories—with fun. To be silent same as barren: no different than exposed. Silence as disclosure, risk of discovery of our hidden yet familiar murk. Incessant conversation, conversely, a haven of still.

Yet silence, perhaps & in fact, is acknowledgment of infirmity of spoken word, empty talk. What would have emerged if every-day-every-hour-every-where Eliot spoke. Onset of Prufrock because Eliot practiced quiet in spoken world. Because Eliot observed—curt—words of sufficiency emerged as poem. Silence in world, internal monologue, equals poem.

Ay, Johnny. It's okay to be quiet—there's no great matter. It is not too late. I write to you, still, speak to you still. We are good, still good, & we are still. Nothing need move. No mouth, no thin strip of lip. Nothing must indicate how now we know that empty means filled.

&

Intentionally left blank.

&

In terms of setting day-to-day aspirational yet attainable goals, entering "Well Child Waiting Room" vs. "Sick Child Waiting Room" at pediatrician's office is set as plausible goal.

&

In terms of setting of story, this story is set in Bogotá & Miami. When story gets pulled toward Guayaquil, resistance emerges. Because of this immediate, ignorant resistance, I, having no knowledge of Guayaquil upon which to base any legitimate form of resistance, consider South America's resistance to itself.

South America's resistance to itself is real. Venezuelan resistance to Colombian. And vice-a-versa. Chilean resistance to Argentinean. And vice-a-versa. Colombian resistance to Ecuadorian. Uruguayan resistance to Paraguayan. Generalized resistance to Bolivian. Resistance to Guayaquil. Knowing nothing whatsoever of Guayaquil.

Wheretofrom continental self-resistance comes. Colonial past, perhaps. Unclear. But enemy was common, was same: Old World nations of Portugal & Spain.

Is South America's ease for self-disdain simply a quest for easy competition, selection of defeatable opponents, to engage a winnable battle. Europe, Asia and North America belong to other leagues. African struggles too similar to South American ones. The only point of comparison, of competition, is us. Us vs. us. (Why not us & us.) Comparison so as to undermine. Slightly better is better, no matter how slight.

Miami & Bogotá & Guayaquil. I position each name upon a single parallel line.

&

In terms of chronology of story, of progression, of specific sequence of events, the succession is this:[13]

---

13 Spoiler alert.

- Parents notice seizure of boy
- Parents take boy to hospital
  - Seizures during day reach at least eight per day
  - Seizures last no more than five seconds each
  - Seizures are laughter, conscious, a need to lean back
  - Night seizures too mild to gain notice, if occurring
- Boy spends three days in hospital
  - Boy gets various tests and scans and doctor visits in hospital
  - EEG is deemed clear; MRI deemed unclear
  - White Doctor assigned as local neurologist
- Boy emerges from hospital
- Parents seek out alternative witch doctors of Bogotá
- Parents update pediatrician
- Nelly, beloved local Reiki worker, recommends oracle book
- Boy's diet changes, habits, too
  - No sugar
  - No wheat
  - No dairy
  - Nothing from the sea
  - No electronics held in hands
- Parents collect medical records, begin medical clinical process of second opinion
  - Perform additional bloodwork
- Spring Break Witch Doctor Tour of Bogotá
  - Seizures during day decrease to at least four per day
  - Seizures last no more than five seconds each
  - Seizures are laughter, conscious, a need to lean back
  - Minor night seizures emerge
- Boy is treated for parasites, purged; continues with changes in diet, habits, too

- Follow up consult with White Doctor, first round of DNA results returned. DNA tests are inconclusive: boy has two mutations of uncertain significance
- Boy gets ultra-high fever flu
  - No seizures during flu
- Boy gets eye and ear infection while recovering from ultra-high fever flu
  - No seizures during infections while recovering from flu
- Boy emerges from ultra-high fever flu
  - Day seizures cease after boy emerges from flu
- Onset of intense night seizures, two to three per night
  - Boy sits up, shouts, thrashes in bed
  - Night seizures last ten to fifteen seconds each
  - Night seizures have order, chronology, one each at:
    - 2–3 am
    - 4–5 am
    - 6–7 am
- Boy returns to school after flu, physically weakened, night seizures reduce his quality of sleep
- Follow-up round of witch doctors in Bogotá
  - At Elsa's office, consult with Cuban Doctor with Russian machine based in Guayaquil
- Day seizures return. Night seizures continue
  - Night seizures magnify, almost thirty seconds in duration
- Insurance approves second opinion
- Parents engage second opinion
  - At same time parents start treatment with Dr. Bravo, local witch doctor who believes he can cure son
- Boy starts medication approved by witch doctors
- Seizures are gone within twenty-four hours of initiating medication
  - At same time Dr. Bravo says boy is clear of seizures

- Maternal family wine company run by mother is sold
- Boys strength returns, with it, his impulsive, aggressive behavior
  - Dietary changes continue
  - Sessions with Dr. Bravo
- Meanwhile parents initiate third online opinion
- Third opinion concurs with diagnosis of second opinion
- Baby Anaya dies
- Parents opt for coastal city of Guayaquil
- Guayaquil doctor unable to treat boy due to heightened electrical activity in boy's brain
- Parents return home with boy

&

In terms of word choice of story, alongside theory of a helpful God, there is theory of language whose compartmentalized thinking I like. Semiotics, like God, is useful, so I reach for & apply. O, God: o, language: o, boy.

Ideas, notions, impressions work together within the mind to wrench the mind into the world of things. Things that have names. Names that are words.

"It" is happening. "It" is seizure. Okay. But before "it" lands on a mouth, on a page, "it" already exists. The event, the moment—that real world happening of "it," the hyperactive neurons, excess of electrical signal in brain— already exists.

Here, I drew "it" for us—

To use the terms of semiotics, disproportionate voltage in right frontal lobe is the signified and can be referred to like this —on March 27, boy had six seizures, six "its," six events,

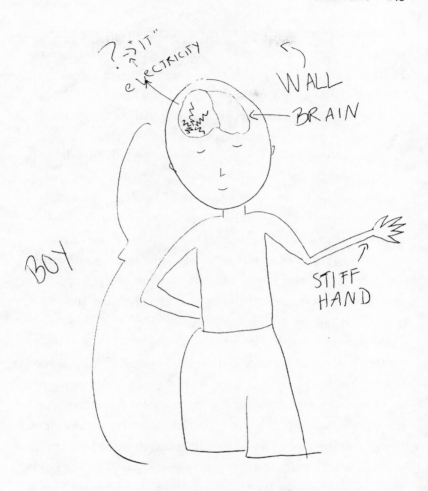

six happenings, six momentary lapses, six absences of physical selfcontrol, six idiopathic near fallings. If you ask: what did boy have. I answer: "it." Six times "it." Six times, the signified.

To write about six seizures I have to use words: I have no other choice. I must use these words, words you and I both know. How else can I tell you there were six seizures on such and such date. I don't paint, I don't sculpt, I don't spin clay into pots. I exercise words, words that may mean more things, or fewer things, than seizure, to you. Lapse, event, happening. Falling sickness. They, these words, may represent something else to you than to me, because you are you, not me.

"Seizure" is unreliable, erratic as word, as are all words. "Seizure." To you it could mean: body fallen to floor crooked as poltergeist vs. to me it means: spasm of singular boy leaning and laughing.

The moment I write "it" down, "it" becomes the signifier. The signifier of the signified. Together, the signifier and the signified form a sign. Signified as event, signifier as term, converged into sign upon the real world. The sign is a summary, a construction built by the perception then naming of actual object that is. Our perception, our naming, yours and mine, into word, haphazardly pinned down.

Semiotics is helpful because it confines.

Boy has seizure. Seizure, is it. Yes—seizure it is. It is laughter. It is nothing. It is something. It is freaky shit. It happens each day, several times each day. It did not happen before it happened. It is idiopathic. It is both electric & magnetic. It is both clinical & medical. It is both symptom & diagnosis. It may also be prognosis. It is both lamp & light. It may be related to pathogens in boy's body. It may be related to structure of boy's brain. It may be triggered by bad diet, electronic devices. It is short lasting. It does not end. It is a condition to life. It is real. It is happening.

There's more, though. Now, there is more. "It" evolves. For "it" is also all the ways "it" enters & departs, the ways "it" forces me to talk, to say, to explain, to request, to employ terms & words to attempt to fathom, to fasten, to trap, what in fact is happening to boy.

What I know: Boy has seizure. "It" is seizure. "Seizure" is a giggling fit. Episodic. Rigorous. All-encompassing. Mild. Obliterating. *Unheimlich* as fax.

&

In terms of soundtrack of story, there are songs that are now the songs of seizure. Boy & his love of music continue to be. In car, boy demands we play his songs. On high rotation: 'Happier' by Marshmello and Bastille. 'Fade' by Allan Walker. 'In My Feelings' by Drake.[14] Always these three songs when boy in car.

Husband and I try to assert our authority by usurping song selection. Husband tells me to play Chicane. Because of boy's love of Allan Walker, its devised electro sci-fi melodic beat, play Chicane. Other times husband asks for Cuban folk music. Ibrahim Ferrer, Eliades Ochoa, Compay Segundo: nostalgia unspooled. Husband sings because husband has good Cuban ballad singing voice. Husband whistles. Husband sings. Despite: we three in car usually means it is a doctor visit ride.[15]

When I make it my turn, I'll put on an Indie cover. Give me

---

14 Boy, when boy is in loving good singing mood, sings to me: "Mimi do you love me; are you riding; say you never ever leave me." A derivation of chorus of Drake's song: "Kiki do you love me…"

15 When Nina Real in car she demands, invariably, soundtrack for *Charlie and The Chocolate Factory* composed by Danny Elfman for Tim Burton. Sometimes she wants the character suites: Veruca Salt, Violet Beaureagarde, Mike Teavee. But, invariably, she wants the Main Title suite. Music that accompanies the initial chocolate-making scenes. Music to launch a Burton children's movie with Johnny Depp & Helena Bonham Carter. Dark chocolate music. Melodic spookiness, offness. Characteristic uncanniness.

pop but give it soft. Desolate & soft, my pop. I go off record one day. Play a song that I aim at husband. Because husband has just sung, has just whistled with his Cuban music voice, I say, it is my turn. I play 'Idilio.' Not the original 1993 version by Willie Colón. Willie Colón, of millions-of-salsa-records-sold, Puerto Rican from The Bronx. But a newer version, one by Colombian signer Fonseca.

This is one of my favorite songs, I tell boy. Tell so husband Nelson David will hear. Will want to know why.

Husband asks why.

Because when I heard it, I wasn't together with your dad. We had been together but at that moment we were not. And I heard the song and even though I wasn't together with your dad, I sent it to him. And because I sent it to him, I knew I loved your dad.

And it is so. I sent husband song because of husband's love for Willie Colón. Willie, not Cristóbal; Colón, not Wonka. I sent song because I wanted husband back. And it worked.

I like that, says husband, whistling to song.

Such a small thing to give, that playing of that song. That day in that car with husband & boy. To say to husband: *remember when I sent you that song.* To say: *I sent you that song because I wanted this so.* Such a small thing to give, but at that moment, that instant, it felt big. Big because scarce: scarce because scare: scare because care.

The soundtrack of seizure is tight with give.

&

In terms of medical, clinical story, it is important to know the difference between medical & clinical. To know, be able to write in my own words—not just think I know—the meaning of the following words, presented and prepared as sets, as couples, couplets of terms: prognosis vs. diagnosis; incidence vs. prevalence; attenuation vs. healing; disease vs. disorder; accept vs. adapt; patient vs. patient.

Ah, the listicle—

1. Clinical vs. Medical
   a. Clinical: quantify through observe, scan, exam. Blood/work. Body on paper. Green numbers on the screen of a hospital's fawn-colored machine. The harvesting of facts from patient unwell. Not: reading of what records mean.
   b. Medical: not medicinal. Not heal, not uproot, not deracinate disease. To handle: doctor as verb. Bad root, rooted in place. Business not of health, but of prescriptions for the body unwell. Remediate.

2. Prognosis vs. Diagnosis
   a. Prognosis: medical vision of future based on clinical view of present and past. How will body unwell live if body unwell survives. Survival often requires substance inserted. Substance inserted improves perfection of bodily life, and so expectancy of it. As in, what to expect from your body, your life.
   b. Diagnosis: identification of how a body is unwell. A conclusion, not to be confused with conclusive. A word for the visuals of what. Not a pit to quarry, not how, not why. Just this—or that.

3. Incidence vs. Prevalence
   a. Incidence: number of new cases of disease that emerge in a given period of time. Rate of onset. Statistical

measure of risk. Extent of odds: my odds, your odds of fall.

b. Prevalence: how many now. Not how many new. How many suffer now. How widespread. Numerical measure of is. Incidentally, the global prevalence of epilepsy is this: strewn fifty million people wide.

4. Attenuation vs. Heal

a. Attenuation: reduction of intensity. Applicable to medical, clinical condition, to disease. *What you want is attenuation*: this, an older doctor friend says. Attenuation of severity of disease. Attenuation of erratic electrical signals of brain. Not to fathom, to distinguish, to restore.

b. Heal: what I want. Heal is not a word hospital doctors use. Not in terms of epilepsy. To treat, to control, to diagnose, to prognose, to medicate: to attenuate. Not cure, nor mend. Sometimes childhood epilepsy goes away. In terms of epilepsy, heal is offered as this: from whence it came, disease leaves, absconds, burns away.

5. Disease vs. Disorder

a. Disease: external affectation turned internal: infection, parasite, virus that renders body ill. Of cause generally known. Originally limited to factually, systemically, literally sick. [sic!] Expanded however to include ailments of the emotional body, the impressionable mind. Summary: symptomatic affectation of the day, or its parts.

b. Disorder: may result from disease. Epilepsy is disorder. Seizure is condition. Seizure is sign. Seizure is symptom. Seizure is disorder. Sign of something further. But also:

sign in and of itself. What is wrong is order. Tough to say what else, exactly, turned amiss.[16]

---

16 In reading about the medical usage of the words "disease" vs. "disorder" I came across this extract, which is particularly revealing regarding the general population's relationship with the words themselves—"The International League Against Epilepsy (ILAE) is an important source of guidance for health professionals when it comes to epilepsy. Their latest recommendation that epilepsy should no longer be called a "disorder," but a "disease" has though caused controversy. The ILAE contends the change will improve epilepsy's image. Some clinicians and other organizations fear the change may not though be accepted by patients as in common parlance "disease" can be associated with "contagiousness"/"infection." To allow practicing clinicians to make informed judgements about what language they use, we completed the first study to assess the preferences of those with epilepsy and significant others and explore if any of their characteristics were associated with preference. Via epilepsy interest groups and associations in England, Wales, Scotland and the Republic of Ireland, 971 patients and significant others were surveyed. Participants identified which of four labels for epilepsy ("disorder," "illness," "disease," "condition") they favoured and rated each using a Likert-scale. Patients' median age was 39; 69% had experienced seizures in the prior year. "Condition" was favoured by most patients (74.3%) and significant others (71.2%). Only 2.2% of patients and 1.2% of significant others chose "disease"; it received a median Likert-rating indicating "strongly dislike." Multinomial logistic regression found it was not possible to reliably distinguish between participants favouring the different terms on the basis of demographics. The ILAE's position is at odds with what most patients and carers want..." https://www.ncbi.nlm.nih.gov/pubmed/28294303

6. Accept vs. Adapt
   a. Accept: to say, okay. To say, so what. Boy has seizures. So what.
   b. Adapt: adapt is easier if first accept. If first, imperfection named and admitted within rituals, routine of life. (Epilepsy: so what!) We can swing and slide, but let's avoid the monkey bars, for now, in today's life.

7. Patient vs. Patient
   a. Patient: body unwell who launches clinical medical process to elicit diagnosis of disorder/disease hoping for cure but who may receive instead prognosis, attenuation via insertion of substance, medication.
   b. Patient: body unsettled able to sip coffee, breathe, stitch together, wait. Symptomatic hope, or is it faith.

&

In terms of unlikely story, on the plane ride back from Bogotá, back from our Spring Break 2019 Witch Doctor Tour of Bogotá, I sit next to Dr. Camilo Cruz who sees me writing like madwoman on plane and remarks on my remarkable madwoman typing skills. I cease attempting to record every significant second of my days in Bogotá with boy and chat to this stranger sitting to my right.

Stranger is nuclear physicist who has written thirty-six self-help/empowerment books & one collection of stories, per the persistent nudging of his friend, one Isabel Allende. Allende who tells him he must do literary MFA to write literary words in addition to words of self-help. She recommends MFA writing program at Colombia's National University. Yes, *La Nacional*. Same MFA where I took class on Freud.

Same MFA I began but failed, halfway, to complete.

Dr. Camilo Cruz and I had many of the same professors, same classes: Azriel Bibliowicz's legendary class on *Ulysses*. Azriel, married to Colombian artist Doris Salcedo, of Tate Modern, multiple international museum solo exhibit and retrospective fame. Joe Broderick, Australian by birth, and his legendary class on Beckett. Dr. Cruz, Camilo, is so friendly. He knows all professors by first name.

I never finished that MFA, I say.

Dr. Cruz is not surprised. *It's hard to know what to do with it,* he says. *Azriel always wondered how many of his students would write afterwards. They cancelled it, you know.*

No way. In the end, it was the bathrooms that were a problem for me. They were revolting. And also Che Guevara. I got tired of everywhere the graffiti of Che. Finally, I revolted.

Ha. Yes. La Nacional is a strange place. Joe finally quit because they wouldn't give him an office with sufficient light.

Ha. Wow. Joe seemed sacrificially communist, too. Did you ever write a book for the MFA.

I did, book of stories. But it was too hard. My other books, my teaching books, come fast, come easy. I just finished another one. It is called Storytelling. *It's about how world's great leaders, great entrepreneurs, are first & foremost great storytellers.*

Though not a writer of it, Dr. Cruz is lover of poetry, a reader of it. Poetry is our way in. Into each other. He tells me his most famous book is called *Once Upon a Cow* and is about settling for nothing but success. Clearly in need of nothing but success, I settle into self-help chatter of self-help guru sitting to my right on plane—

Basically, you just cannot blame your parents. Or anything/anyone else. No use blaming self. What you think is not what you know. It's just what you think. The chatter within. Thinking is not good because it keeps you from knowing because when you think, you think you know. So you don't rethink, you just continue. You don't nudge. So you don't emerge. Excellence as derivative of collision. Remarkable as subversion of day-to-day pre-package presentation of self as only self. Onset of change as spark of wake.

Dr. Cruz becomes my best airplane friend. We exchange emails. We are going to have good coffee and talk Latin American books. Really at some point we are. He will order my book of poems. I will order his book of cows.

All my books, he says, *start with poem. Single same poem. Drives my editor nuts. But books sell anyway.*

Poem's name is "En paz" (At Peace) by Amado Nervo, Mexican modernist poet. Incidentally, his poem is published on the same year as my Prufrock is published: 1915.[17]

Eliot, Nervo, Jonathan, Lispector, Kipling, Har Dyal, Elsa, Nelly, Sergio, Elizabeth, Vet, Warhol, Cruz, Columbus, et al. My plots thicken. My pulse quickens. As I go, I deploy certain, real world pursuit of non-incidental onset of un-sick boy.

Below, first two stanzas of Amado's poem, poem which lives in reduced, quotational form within each of Dr. Cruz's thirty-six self-help books—

Porque veo al final de mi rudo camino
que yo fui el arquitecto de mi propio destino;

---

17   'The Love Song of Alfred J. Prufrock' first appeared in *Poetry: A Magazine of Verse* in 1915.

que si extraje las mieles o la hiel de las cosas,
fue porque en ellas puse hiel o mieles sabrosas:
cuando planté rosales, coseché siempre rosas.

&

Because in the end of my rough ride,
I realize that I've been the architect of my life;

that if I extracted honey or gall,
it's because I put forth honey or gall:
when I planted rosaries, I always harvested roses.

7

Batter my heart, three-person'd God, for you
As yet but knock, breathe, shine, and seek to mend (John Donne)

We are in April. Eliot's cruelest month. The month of thaw, of wet earth, of rebirth. Birth hurts, breaks the womb, cracks the ground, maims comfortable flesh with flow of new, self-warmed blood. Is this what Eliot means. Is this what he means by cruel. Spring who ruins Winter. Ruinous Spring. Winter, who just wants to be. Blue, white, grey, grim—but be.

On the April new moon, on this month's blackened, nascent advent of moon, we have follow-up with White Doctor. We understand nothing of what he says, this doctor in white who speaks dark as absent lamplight. Nor do we grasp anything of what he leaves out.

What we are certain of is this: boy has two Messi's in his windowless presence.

We talk a lot. We talk a lot about how we are still not on medication. We talk about some of the alternative methods we are trying, the no sugar, no dairy, no gluten. The no electronics. The heavy metal testing, the zinc, the selenium, the magnesium, the B complex. The positive Epstein-Barr. The parasite. We leave out Doctor Carmona & his biomagnetism. We leave out Eli & her Vet. We leave out Elsa & her Guayaquil. We certainly leave out Sergio & his Hamer Points. We do not tell of our only happy stories.

When the White Doctor speaks, he speaks in reverse. He tells us he went back to boy's EEG, taken during hospital stay one month ago. White Doctor reread EEG & EEG was indeed not clear. Was unclear. Is opposite of clear. He tells us that he also went back to boy's MRI. That this MRI was indeed, instead, clear. Is clear. Clear, clear. The exact converse of what we were told a month ago, exact inverse of what our printed medical clinical story, our records, our history shows.

Is this what Eliot means by April, by "dull root". White Doctor is quiet. It is our turn to utter.

Why does MRI written printed report we receive after three days in hospital read that there is something on right frontal lobe, I say.

MRI technicians want to help us doctors, he says. *They know we are so desperate to try and figure things out that they sometimes are overeager. They overreach. They give us something that is not there so that we can give answers. But the MRI is clear. I was, however, able to pick up on definite seizure activity on the EEG. The EEG is not clear. Boy had seizures. Has. Seizures.*

So what does this mean for boy's future.

You mean his prognosis.

Yes. Okay. His prognosis.

He can have a fully normal life, but I strongly suggest medication. Once a person has seizures there is an increased likelihood that they can suffer a severe one. This is something no parent wants to witness. Something nobody wants to witness period. Also, there's an epilepsy camp you can send him to this summer. I can give you a flyer for it.

Epilepsy camp. Send him to epilepsy camp. He is six.

You could go too. You can meet other families whose kids have epilepsy. Other kids like him. Other families like yours.

What about the genetic test. Did you get results.

Yes I got the results.

Okay.

White Doctor does not want to talk about DNA. White Doctor does not know how to talk about DNA. Granted it is hard to talk about DNA. But we are parents with a boy with one-month-old epilepsy waiting for an answer, throbbing for an answer, and he is our doctor. Our White Doctor with long-awaited DNA results and we've heard him talk about epilepsy camp and medication and say nothing, nothing at all, about the results, which are, on whatever level, literally, technically, verbally, printed—results.

What do the results say. When can we pick up.

We only ran a panel of seventy epilepsy genes. There are over two thousand known epilepsy-related genes. Dysplasia alone has two hundred known related genes. He has mutations on two of the seventy genes we tested. None appear to be hereditary. Although we cannot say for sure. One appears to be suspicious. But we, all of us, we all have two copies of each gene, and he only has mutations on one of each of the copies. So, of the pair, he has one mutation, one normal gene. We can run a triad DNA. This means take samples from parents and from boy, from the three of you. Run a full panel of the two thousand epilepsy related genes for all three of you. This will help determine if mutations are hereditary or not.

You can pick up test we ran here at hospital in a week or so, he says. *We will have results printed for you in week or so. It will take some time. Not today. In a week or so. You need to sign a release first. That you can do today. We'll run it through the hospital's records department. But, be aware, when you receive them, results may be difficult to understand.*

Husband and I say nothing because we understand nothing. I wonder, internally, why we didn't run triad DNA test a month ago in hospital, understanding, comprehending, grasping only that what we are handed is not results, but another wait. Four to six more weeks of wait. For results. Everything in medical clinical world takes four to six weeks. Then the results: results that are delivered as if they were a gift. A favor. Like it is not our right to know because we don't know enough to know, to understand. Like doctor will not explain because to explain to us is to disburse unwarranted breath. To waste breath.

Give boy medication. Check out epilepsy camp, doctor says, standing up.

Are mutations linked to any other disease, condition, disorder, anything degenerative.

Not that we know of. There is one that is suspicious. Let's do the triad. Let's get you and your husband's DNA under a microscope. For now, start the Keppra. Call if you see anything odd.

Prognosis is medication. Future is medication. To give boy drug, to insert substance, continues to feel like giving up.

&

Boy gets flu. Mid-April, mid-cruel. One week before Easter. Six weeks after stay at hospital with "Terminal" name. Two weeks after 2019 Spring Break Witch Doctor Tour of Bogotá. One week after White Doctor visit to obtain reversed reading of adverse results.

Boy gets flu. Fever begins to swell on last day of his purgative. Albendazole, prescribed by Vet, doctor not of humans but of animals that live in houses, pets.

The dosage of Albendazole is this: one on day one, one on day five, one on day fifteen. On day fifteen, two weeks after Colombia, boy gets flu.

Boy gets flu. Last day of purgative. Boy loses between three point five to four pounds due to flu. Boy is already very low in weight. Roughly speaking boy's loss of weight equates to ten percent of his body mass, ten percent reduction of mass of boy burned off as fever into adjacent, empty space.

The fevers of flu for the first five nights:

- 103.4
- 105.3
- 105.1
- 104.8
- 104.5

In brief duration of life, boy has never had fever as high, as dry as this. Boy is asleep all day. He sleeps. He burns. He senses, imagines, cold. He is furnace of parched brittle heat who quivers with cold. He does not eat. He is sleep. He is not life-awake, not lift. It is purgatory, it is sink. Faint arid aura mist. Life as state of in-between.

Boy does not have seizures while boy has flu. Not even with the high fever, fever being a a principal trigger of seize. All seems off. How is it possible for seizure disease with ultra-high fever to cease.

We visit pediatrician twice in one week. *It is flu*, she says, insists, confirms. *Go home. It is just the flu. Just. The flu. Relax.*

Seizure is better than extreme high fever of flu, we, husband & I, say. Seizure is better than no seizures despite extreme high fever of flu, then why is boy not having seizures if boy so weakened by feral fever of flu, than wondering, unknowing, gauging when it is time for another hospital trip: should we pack bags. Should we pop open Keppra, measure substance, insert. What is going on with fiendishly feverish seizure-free boy.

We, husband and I, take turns sleeping with boy. One night on, one night off. Flu lasts ten nights. Chest of boy fully constricted. Barren, aching cough that does not let boy sleep. Lack of sleep another major trigger of seizures.

Yet. No seizures—not one. Not even a suspicious twitch, an exaggerated sneeze, during flu.

I write Vet and Elizabeth, Eli, my good witch at the heart of my Bogotá. Tell them of flu. Describe it all in detail. Of last day of Vet's parasite purgative being same as first day of flu.

It is curative crisis, Eli says. *This is part of healing. First, it must get worse.*

Now pediatrician is telling us that he developed an ear infection and eye infection, both, all while boy is beaten by flu, ravaged by cough, I say.

Aconitum napellus, says Vet. *Homeopathic remedy for sudden onset of fever with dry skin.*

For now, cease the belladonna, he says. *Belladonna works for fevers that break out in sweat. Aconitum is for fevers that are dry. Give him ten to twelve pellets a day of aconitum for now.*

Shall I give him antibiotics, antiviral. The pediatrician says we need, boy needs. For infections of ear and of the eye. But antibiotics weaken immune system, hinder ability to battle virus, parasite, whatever it is he has.

Yes, says Eli. *Yes*, says Vet. *Give him antiviral antibiotic antihistamine inhalations & homeopathy. Give him all. He can take it. He requires it. Give it all.*

He is so thin, I say. *So thin.*

Give it time, Eli says. *From this he will recover. I have to say. I like what I see.*

Curative crisis. Total body collapse into renewed health. We believe a change is coming, has come. A cellular molecular battle overcome. Could it be.

&

On a Monday, the eleventh morning since onset of flu, we reemerge—take boy to school. Boy is weak but begging for school. Wants to play soccer at soccer class Monday at school. We go. We take. We walk, at this instant, seizure free. Ten days times twenty-four hours, not a single convulsion. It is day eleven. We wade forward. Aware of eleven. Ambitious eleven.

Teacher, remarkably remarkable, greets boy, gathers, encircles, amasses him in.

Oh my, she says, *but how his arms & legs are thin*.

&

We have not come full circle. We have perhaps begun to loosely draw circle. Not closed, nor delimited, the ring of round. Yet, we are thickly encircled. Radially affixed. Whatever the progress, its lack, the drawing of shape, the shape of drawing, although uncertain, is bound. Outline compass, we advance as sphere, go nowhere, orbit as sphere.

&

On second night of flu, when fever surpasses one hundred & five for first time in boy's life. We bathe boy at one o'clock in the night.

Don't turn on lights, I say to husband, within dark bathroom. *Boy does not like bright light when he is just recently awake*.

Okay, husband says. Even though husband likes bright bathroom light even at one o'clock in the night.

Boy with fever of one hundred and five speaks: *light creates heat*.

Boy sits in shower and allows himself, in the dark, to be cooled, to be bathed, to be doused with water like a furious flame.

&

For a day. Did I say. One day after flu. Boy is seizure free. Did   I say.

Have I mentioned this. Seizure-free-boy. I cup Vet's small clear moonstone drops in my hands. Could it be. Could it. Be. Memory of disease. Reversed. Boy's nervous wreck, restored. Curative crisis a conquest of onset.

Remarkably, unremarkable boy, returned. For a day. Or so. We believe. Believe with weak faith, with faint hope, unease.

Epilepsy of boy: happening of it: no more. Could. It. Be.

The moonstone drops of our vet:

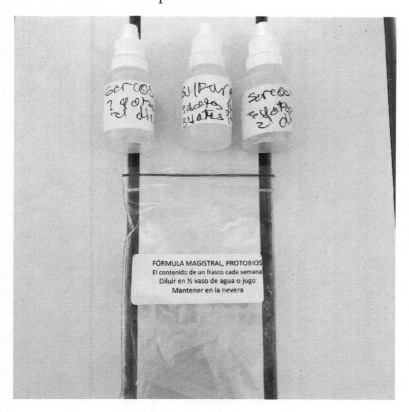

&

It could be. But it is not. Not so. What it is: new pattern: new
load.

Flu ends, then,   night seizures   blossom   burgeon.

&

Marian apparitions are the name given to idiopathic appear-
ances, emergences of the Virgin Mary. To her miraculous rev-
elations. Marian apparitions are myriad. But one of the most
famous is this: Virgin Mary appears before an Aztec Catholic
convert named Juan Diego in 1591, speaking Juan Diego's language, just outside of Mexico City. She is a Mexican Virgin.
With native tongue & native skin speaking to native son. She is
Virgin of Guadalupe.

Three times she appears to Juan Diego, tells him to go to
the Bishop and ask Bishop to build a church at site of her apparition.[18] Three times the Bishop disbelieves. Three times the
Bishop asks for a sign. Three times Juan Diego goes back. Back
to the apparition. But on the fourth day, when he is supposed
to go back, Juan Diego stands the Virgin up. His uncle is sick,
dying. Juan Diego tends to his uncle.

Virgin will not be stood up. She goes, she finds Juan Diego
on path to sick uncle's house. Virgin asks Juan Diego why he did
not seek her, pray to her, implore her, entreat her. In his time
of need, why not beseech Her. Then: in time of need. Virgin
says—

Am I not here with you, I, who am your Mother.

Myriad accounts of Virgin of Guadalupe have this single

---

18 (Go tell it on the mountain!)

singular phrase in common. *Am I not here with you, I, who am your Mother*. After Virgin says this, Virgin provides Juan Diego with sign for Bishop to believe. A cape with her image miraculously, idiopathically, embossed. Bishop believes. An altar is built, altar turns into church, church becomes basilica. A basilica that converts into a Catholic pilgrimage site, one of world's most populous. Forty thousand people can fit inside Guadalupe's basilica for mass. Estimates reckon twenty million pilgrims visit the Virgin of Guadalupe at her basilica each year.

Twenty million people journey to a unique here, a precise here. To pray, ask, beseech. Of Her, who is here.

Twenty million material bodies per year in search of I. In search of I, who am here. In search of I, who am your Mother.

And is your Mother not here.

&

On Easter Sunday, I remove Nina Real from her crib at 9:30 am. Nina Real who is able to sleep adolescent-like even though she is three.

Nina Real, I say. *It is time to try to make it to church at your school. See your friends. Give thanks. Wake up. Let's eat. We are late.*

She does not move.

Nina, I say.

I am not Nina. Woof. Woof.

Woof, woof. Come on little puppy, wake up.

As child I did not pretend to be dog like Nina Real, but I slept like Nina Real. I slept until I was allowed to sleep by adult. Three of the traits that defined me as child: excessive sleep, absence of eating, excessive book. Three of the traits that define Nina Real: excessive sleep, pretending to be other, excessive talk. Three traits that define boy: excessive physical sport, absence of eating, excessive mind. Boy got absence of eating. Girl got excessive sleep. This is how DNA works: it unhooks its double helix form so as to replicate, segment by segment, unzipped. Female DNA combines with male DNA, fragment by fragment, unhinged. This trait from her, that trait from him. No, not that trait. Leave that one behind. Or dormant. For now.

Who decides who gets what. How. Who decides, or is it what. Is it what who decides who. Incidentally, why. Where from comes excessive physical sport if father and mother have none. There is an uncle though, brother of father, who expressed excessive sport. Is it a trait dormant in father to be actuated in renewed present time by boy. Will no child be the child to receive my beloved definitive attribute of excessive book.

Or, is excessive book perhaps now transfigured, evolved, into Nina Real pretending to be other, pretending to be dog. Because excessive, inquisitive, mind of boy seems, to me, not to be trait of excessive book transmuted: not escapist enough, rather, rooted in science, in structure, in the infrastructure of his world.

Absence of eating: in terms of evolution, it makes no sense. Eating is survival. Not eating is risk added, of disease, virus, bacteria, fungus, parasite, seizure entering body, entering DNA, overtaking, attacking, pilfering strength. If DNA wants only to replicate, to survive, why not leave that trait behind. Unless.

Unless there is more. More to the way of want of bureaucratic nucleotide.

&

Night seizures have general, temporal pattern. They occur at midnight, three am, six am. They last thirty seconds to a minute. Day seizures rarely last longer than five seconds.

In my own words, this is what night seizure looks like—

Boy's breathing contracts, quickens, becomes audible. Boy's breathing as aura of onset. Boy speaks. Speaks loudly, shouts. Soccer sagas on repeat. Messi scores a hat trick. Another one! Of Russia eliminating Spain from the last World Cup. Speaks of nonsense, of not killing his head. Names Pokémon characters. Speaks of Ronaldo, of not Ronaldo. Shouts: no, not Ronaldo.

While boy shouts he sits up. Left arm stiff at right angle, so taut it agitates. Legs extend & stiffen, ossify. Eyes open into the hollow slit of an old mailbox. After, a noise like whine, like wail, then chuckle, cackle, chortle. Not slender giggles of day but remarkable bout of abdominal laughter. Rotund snickers, with intensity of whirling but stationary wheel. Boy, spun by spindle, turned into axle, twisted by torque.

During seizures boy never wakes. He shouts, sits, stiffens, moans, laughs, demands water, drinks, gulps, swallows, then bores down to continue sleep. All the while: non-responsive, nonexistent, absent.

After three am fit I don't sleep. My body, its mind, ajar. My mind, its body, agape. I hold vigil for the six am shift, await awake boy's six am howl.

&

Elsa writes often to ask of boy. *How is boy.*

We don't know. Better in a way. Only seizing at night, we say. *But seizing hard, seizing loud.*

At end of month Cuban doctor comes to Bogotá, she says. *Bring boy to Cuban doctor at end of month in Bogotá. Think about it. Piénsenlo.*

&

On Easter Sunday, a few hours before I wake Nina Real, three Catholic churches & three hotels are bombed in Colombo, Sri Lanka. Husband and I read about it, learn about it, at the end of the day, a warm, perky, beach-ready Easter Sunday in Miami.

With the reading of news at night, we slacken, submerge into sadness, empathy of abundant tragedy. Our mostly-only-happy Easter Day, night seizure depletion despite, sugar-ban-during-Easter-egg-hunt-brawls despite, withdraws. At night, in bed, we see images emerge: the details. The children gone. Always, I read about the children gone. The parents with young children gone. It is only the human loss details I read. The sudden absence I consume. Not the details of why, of how. What isis claims or does not claim, I skim, shelve. It is happening. The bombs happened. It stopped. The bombs stopped. The small children, the young parents, gone. It is this information I labor to learn, absorb. The aftermath, the algebra of after the bombs stop, the subtraction, divisions, fractions— the mathematics of loss. Within these numbers, these crooked equations, encapsulated, is absence. I am drawn by, drawn into this geometry of abrupt, size-less demise.

Compulsively, in the days that follow, I continue to read life stories of those killed. The number of dead, 253. Not 249. Not 252. Not 254. Exactly 253. One fifth of dead are children. Around fifty. Do I know fifty children well. Yes, certainly. I know so many. That many. But I only know one who died. Lionel. Fifty times Lionel. Fifty times the hurt, the absence, the face that is small, soft and squishy then gone. The violence of irreversibly gone.

Too much information contained inside, within, the folds of facts. Facts that are facts, numerical markers, descriptors of death. How many. How old. How many from single family. A British family, two out of two children gone, mother gone, father remains. A Sri Lankan set of grandparents, son, daughter-in-law, three children, gone. A local mother, husband, two teenage children gone. A Danish family on Easter holiday having breakfast, three out of four children gone. I think of people I know with four children. The few. I think of three out of four.

$$\frac{3}{4} \qquad \frac{2}{4} \qquad \frac{1}{4}$$

I think of my one out of my two. Of what is at stake with my one who is sick, unwell, seizing, convulsive: one epileptic out of two, my two, two of whom I can still hold. I consider the numbers that are used to explain the ones who survive. Of survive. Of "survive" as being half of a whole word. To live is not the same as to survive. What survives. The mother with one out of four. The grandmother with son, daughter-in-law, grandchildren gone. Does she survive. Who is she when in the aftermath she is the integer, the single statistic of live.

Two out of my two. Two out of two, not the same, despite fractional mathematics, as one out of one.

It is only via the 253 victims of far lands of Colombo that I can cry for the muted thought of possible loss of my one. Loss on foreign land is only loss I allow to expand as emotion that is local, that is mine. Am I sad. I am. I am manifestly, phonetically, audibly sad. I read about the funerals of the children. The half-families. I zoom into the mother's face. I attach until I cannot bear it, become drained of hurt, beset by it—I turn, I jerk, I click, retreat away.

$$\frac{2}{2} \quad \frac{1}{1}$$

Weeks pass, but I return. Return to my mostly sunny Easter Sunday. Return to that instantaneously, unfathomably tragic Easter Day. Is there such a thing as an only happy story, an only happy day. What is this place, this planet, this sphere encircled by life-sustaining sky, gravitas of dirt, of accidental, incidental ash. Of God and lesson and lesson delivered via loss of child.

Is it paltry of me, low of me, to return to news of massive bombs in far-off lands. Is it for tolerable sadness of other that I search for when I search for news of bomb. Do I hunt legitimate sad, removable sad. Sad like bandage of distant bomb on distant face. Sad like life goes on because those who live survive. Sad like survive.

It is only through Colombo's factual actual loss that I grasp—grasp, not grab—that which is mine, that which I have, yet, to hold, that which is mine that is at stake.

No matter how much I read about Colombo, no matter how I dissect the photos of the observable pain of loss, no matter how much I feel the empathy of tragedy rise, I am certain I do not clasp, do not seize, how seismic death of child evolves to become an actual fractional part of planetary life.

&

Mid-April. Mid-cruel. Post-flu. The calendar advances, seizure despite. Time for my twenty-year high school reunion. Seriously. Class of 1999. Husband and I are ready for some form of revelry. For break. For chatter that is talk. We go. In some form, we go.

I see, encounter, good friend Kim. Kim to whom I must tell of boy's epileptic spells. It's a shame to spoil the fun. But Kim is friend with whom I must share.

I tell. She listens. Her husband listens. Her eyes water. She reaches out to grab, to grasp, me.

How often is this happening.

Every day.

Oh my God. How many times.

It got to be six to eight when we first caught it. But now the seizures are only at night. None during the day, lately. We've changed his diet: no sugar, no gluten, no dairy. Lots of supplements. Hardly any electronics. Maybe that's working. But he's having some four seizures every night. So, something's still off.

Oh Ana.

It's okay, I say, I soothe. We are grateful. They aren't Poltergeist *seizures, on the floor, stiff, with eyes rolled back. When they happened during the day, they were laughing seizures. Gelastic seizures they might be called. He would laugh and lean back against something for some five seconds. Now at night they last longer and are way creepier. But there is so much worse. Out there. There is so much worse. One doctor called what boy has le petit mal. This means it is bad, but not too bad. We are working on it. We will figure it out. Or we will have to figure something out. There's the medication, too, which we have not given. Oh Kim, don't be sad.*

I am so sorry, she says. She is sad. She is tearing. She leans into hug me because she is sad. Her face, her aura, her actions are function of sad.

You seem calm, Kim's husband says. *Are you the worrier. Or is your husband. Who is the worrier of your house.*

Ha. I guess he is. In terms of boy's epilepsy, yes, for sure, he is.

Kim is our worrier, he says. *There is a worry quota per household. If one of the two parents fills it up then the other parent does not have to worry. That is something we've figured out. For most things Kim fills our quotient. I only have a few things that it's my turn to worry about.*

Huh. Well then, husband fills most of our health of boy worry quota. Not all of it. But most.

It's a zero-sum game, he shrugs. *The more one parent worries the less the other one has to. Or will. Or probably even can. There really is a limit to the worrying. At least we think so. It sounds, though, like everything will be okay.*

Yeah. Thanks. Maybe not okay. But fine, at least. I really believe that. That we will find a way to adapt and be fine. Husband might not say the same right at this instant. But in your zero-sum worry game equation, on average, probably, we can both agree on fine.

Fine's okay.

Yes. It is. I agree. Fine will have to be okay.

&

A filament of words form within me to ask if DNA is keyboard of source. Alphabet of every story, range of combine, ruler to measure out creation by. Both software and license. An ampersand. &.

We concede: DNA is basic blueprint of life. Nucleotide blocks, elemental code, with which to form. But also inform, deform, mal-form. Inside: genes for conditions that are threat can remain dormant for an entire being's life. Or wake. Awake, alive. Emerge. Set on.

In boy's story, gene for epilepsy awakes alive. Is it a parasite that wakes it up. Is it Epstein-Barr. Strep or Staph. Not the one, but the combination of. Meanwhile, sugar galloping through boy's already invaded, predisposed, blood. Meanwhile, electric devices held by boy's defenseless hands.

Gene for seizure swarms alive, begins to operate, to decide. Gene whose very existence is already a pre-decision, a pre-condition, the result not of replication but of inexplicable, random genetic mutation. Not even of the mother, not even of the father. Not parent, not host. Not them but another architect who resolves, who adopts.

DNA, chance, parents, nature, source. Who is it who concocts. Who formulates story of seizure via mutation buried within firstborn child.

Then, the day-to-day pollution of life. Then, the parent-run family. Then, the microscopic invasion imbalance of life. Then, the electromagnetic assault on life.

Parents: flawed, permissive parents. Permissive parents because of our double-helix-driven day-to-day. Parents who by innate design, by blueprint within their bodies alive, require not only work but personal projects to thrive. Parents who overwork. Who give-in-to-child because of excessive urge for enterprise. Because of the implicit, comes the explicit.

For this family, DNA says, the lesson of seizure is now: a soundtrack on its turntable ready to twirl, a potion in its cauldron commanding a swirl. It is time, now, for this family's ultimate understanding of ultimate reality to conflate. Time to disrupt.

Because of choice, chance.

Here we are. By chance. By choice. By stroke of luck: by code: by omniscient keyboard. We have a chance, a choice. The option to remedy, to heal, to learn.

DNA is both. Within its double-ladder climbs the pre and the post. Free will bound by the possibilities of character and plot. DNA is all. Original, initial intelligence and the slow reveal of experience. The will to will.

Not all iterations of oxygen, hydrogen, nitrogen, phosphorus are deemed alive. Is an oxygen atom in the air that floats outside alive. We say *no*. Why. Because it does not seek to replicate, it merely conjoins, by electromagnetic force, combines. Is oxygen atom inside blood alive. Not in and of itself but, yes, it is incarnate, part of corporeal life.

The will to will. To replicate. To make more intelligent, selfsame life. The instinct to endure, to reproduce, to invoke. As basic as eat, as sex, is pray. As basic as human life is faith. Energetic hope. We are built to search for ultimate source. Even agnosticism acknowledges faith by rebutting it—this vs. that God for which I venture disbelief.[19]

Built to hunt, to hound. Encircled. A journey out that irrevocably, invariably leads home. As prodigal offspring we return. Source within. Source that is spark. Spark that compels oxygen, hydrogen, nitrogen, phosphorus to combine, alive, into strands of DNA that type, tell, foretell story that unfolds as a *bildungsroman*.

&

---

19 It. "It."(It!) Always so difficult to summarize it.

My favorite encounter at twenty-year high school reunion is with Richard F. Richard F. was not friend in high school but became friend during college. Regular lunch companion in college. Companion who brought respite, a source of lunchtime laughter.

Do you remember in college when you spent a year abroad in Russia and had the worst time and the best time ever, I say.

What do you mean.

That you loved Russia except for that family you stayed with. How it was a disaster.

Ha. Oh yeah. A total disaster.

I don't remember the story. But I remember laughing about it. Laughing so much. Remind me the story again.

The host family I was staying with was this older couple, wife and husband. They weren't horrible really. But while I was there the wife discovered that the husband was having a major affair. Then it became a disaster. She kicked him out. I was fully on her side the whole time. Totally on Team Irina.

Ha.

I'd wanted to have this quiet year abroad, reading dense Russian novels, living with an old Russian couple. And instead it was this explosive soap opera. We really just can't get away from our life.

What do you mean.

Well, back then I was going through basically the same thing with my mom. And then I get it again, this time in Russian.

I am certain Richard F. never mentioned his own family drama when he told me story in college. Told me repeatedly because I asked, wanting to laugh, repeatedly. Quiet, translucent Richard F. tells it so well, even if over and over & over again.

Ha. It's true, I say. *We can't get away from our life. I like that. So, what are you up to now.*

We talk. Talk a lot. About what Richard F. is up to now. Job at World Health Organization in Geneva, obtained via years spent working in Africa. *I was painting a house to make some cash,* he says, *and I got a call from a college friend who said he was looking for people to work at an* NGO *in a city I'd never heard of. I said yes without thinking.*

I listen to Richard F. It feels good to listen without desire for interruption, interjection, interpolation. Who cares about my story while Richard F. tells his story. Talk does not feel one-sided, but right-sided. I realize now, twenty literal years later, that I sought out Richard F. to hear his subdued talk. Talk that is unadorned, true, does not take.

I do not offer information on what I am up to now. And Richard F. does not query. It is unnecessary, after all, the telling of my work, my day-to-day. We have no need for talk to be of you & me.

Perhaps, Richard F. intuits all. Spares me the saying, the speaking about, the doingness of unwell boy. We keep it pastel. Halcyon talk that is big because it is not small.

&

Because of night seizures and lack of sleep, I nap. Naps that are collapse. In car I pull over into parking lots. From the highway take an exits to sleep outside Home Depot. I become someone who is late in the morning, rushing to reduce the breadth of late. Yet, still, at times, something wakes me up to write. Thieves time from sorely needed sleep to write. In my brain, inside mind, something says: wake up, write.

Because of night seizures and lack of sleep, I nap. Naps that are collapse. In car I pull over into parking lots. From the highway take exits to sleep at Home Depot. I become someone who is late in the morning, rushing to reduce the breadth of late. Yet, still, at times, something wakes me up to write. Thieves time from sorely needed sleep to write. In my brain, inside mind, something says: wake up, write.

I am so tired. I want so much to sleep. Yet, me, I, the voice of mind, says: wake up. Who calls. Who wakes up. Who summons, who emerges. Who the switch: who the lamplight.

&

Have you talked to Josh, someone says at twenty-year high school reunion.

No. Not yet. Want to. Why.

He's doctor at hospital where you went with boy.

Really.

Yeah, an endocrinologist now.

Really. Wow. A pediatric endocrinologist.

Yeah.

Huh. That's a lot.

&

In the bedroom my thoughts come & go, lingering upon Colombo.

Could it be Colombo, too, like Colombia, named after Columbus. If so, when did Columbus go. Was Columbus somehow first: first to come, first to name. Except Columbus was not first. Never was he first. But when Columbus came: he came to name.

A fortunate thing America earned the name of a cartographer and not of a conqueror. Even if mapmakers, too, came to name, there is a difference in their naming, in their coming. The lines they draw, they draw by finger, not fist. Delineate membranes, trace borders, define the instant land changes hands, changes tongues, becomes threshold, beckons passport.

How thin to draw the line, they must think. How thick. Lines between earth and water: terrestrial auras etched by wrist.

None of this do I bother looking up. All of it mere onset of insomniac dark bedroom where three four five am no sleep. So many thoughts, so many words that traverse mind, the labyrinthine folds of brain, thoughts that surface, that emerge, that come to name.

&

As for Nina Real, she is named after friend I had in and after college. No, not named after, but because of. Nina Friend was girlfriend of my then boyfriend's friend. After amorous relationships ended, Nina Friend and I stayed, remained, friends.

A German girl, Münchenien. Tall, blonde, exulted. She liked to date Latins. We spent a lot of time those first two years straight out of college drinking in her New York apartment. Nina Friend already at high power job working for L'Oréal. Her apartment was big, clean, with a view. She had things of size I felt disqualified to have. Double my physical, material, size, she was munificent, a navel, an exalted, placental prize.

To sit with her in that apartment. Clean, white, with view, drinking wine and food she ordered was to enter womb. I ate and drank and slept. I took. I grew from what was fed. I remember being friend: I loved my Nina Friend: but what was it that I lent.

Last time I saw her was in Munich, Fall 2004. She'd moved back: I visited for Oktoberfest. Met her new boyfriend: Mexican this time. In her apartment, ate, slept, drank again too much.

Half a decade later: messages through social media, emails asking for her address. Where to send the invitation to my wedding. The invitation printed, but, for lack of address, never sent.

What was it about me that made her drop me. Was it my hunger for her mothering. What porcelain rim did our friendship crack. In retrospect, did she regret her give. Realize I was not her babe. That she could pick up the hem of her thick, tartan skirt, and go. And, do I admire her for it. Probably, I do. To retrieve her yield of mother: lend it to another. Enough with Ana Friend.

It is not something I think about often: the terse end of Nina Friend. It is gap. A stillbirth. Synapse with no spark.

&

Hey Josh. How are you. Good to see you. How've you been.

Wow, hi, great to see you, too.

Someone just mentioned you're a pediatric endocrinologist. That's pretty incredible.

Ha. Yeah. Thanks.

You know. We were just at hospital where you work for three days with our kid. Just last month. He has seizures. They are calling epilepsy.

Am so sorry. If you need anything ever I'll give you my number. Please just text me.

Thank you. Well, you know, the truth is we really haven't had a good experience with the hospital, with the doctor we were assigned. No clear message from him. It's really hard to talk to him. To understand what's going on with boy.

You know, neurology is tough. Really tough. That's why I chose endocrinology. With endocrinology it's all a matter of addition and subtraction. If hormones are off, you work the numbers and replace, fix what's off. But with neurology, it's hard, there is so much we don't know still about the brain. I've found a certain kind of person chooses to be a neurologist. It usually doesn't go along with being a very good people person. Even more so with pediatric neurologists. Kids brains aren't even fully formed so that's just messy. Endocrinology never gets so complicated I've found.

Yeah. That's been the case for us for sure. Our doctor is definitely not a people person. He doesn't even try to explain things to us. I mean. Okay. To be fair it can't be easy to talk to families who have kids with epilepsy and not to be able to give them answers.

Yep. I can imagine. Parents hang onto your every word when you're a doctor, sometimes it's just better to say less. The toughest my job will get is I'll have a 4' 10" mom come in and go nuts about why her son won't grow, demanding growth hormones.

Ha. That sounds truly tough.

Not as tough as not being able to tell someone what their kid has. But I worked with a few neurologists a while ago that were good. I've had a few drinks so probably won't remember their names right now. Give me your number though and I'll text you this week. There are some really good ones in town. No reason why you shouldn't be happy with your doctor.

Awesome. Thanks. And how do you like working inside the hospital. It seems like such a complex place. Nothing easy, nothing clear, about it.

I actually just finished an MBA a few weeks ago. Did it because I just needed to understand the business side of things. It all wasn't making sense to me to be honest. The reasons for things in the hospital just didn't make sense. Like there really isn't a concern for health. It's crazy. The system works in favor of other things. The business side of things. I'm still trying to figure it out.

You know. We've been going to a bunch of doctors in Colombia, actually. Not that we have any real answers yet, but it feels like there's a different king of asking going on. Like an actual interest in figuring out the why. With our neurologist here, we feel like he just wants us to medicate and forget about the disease. There's no asking at all.

That's good you are digging. Sometimes doctors in places that have less access to the crazy equipment are better.

What do you mean.

Here we have so much stuff. At the hospital, for example, we have all this insane amount of insanely expensive equipment. There's real pressure to use it. To use it and get what looks like results. But not all of it really works to be honest. In terms of diagnosing, it's like sometimes we just need to think about things instead of testing and testing. But it's real tempting to rely on machines instead of thinking about things.

That's just it. And not only the machines but the medication. The neurologist keeps insisting we give boy Keppra and take him to epilepsy camp.

Epilepsy camp. What's that.

Exactly. Now that we are epilepsy people, we need to be sent away with all the other epilepsy folk. It's bizarre.

Well, let me send you the names of other doctors in town. Are you looking for a second opinion.

We are. We just got approved in fact. Mid-May.

That's really soon. Okay. Good. Yeah. Insurance companies like second opinions. Second opinions, if they catch a misdiagnosis, can save a lot of money.

That makes sense. I guess it is soon. Although. That's another thing. I have to say medical time seems different than normal time. Things that are slow are considered fast in medical time.

Ha. Yep. Totally true.

Well. Here's my number. But already you have helped me. Thank you. So much.

&

An alternate title for this book, one of only casual consideration, is—

Seizure & Other Observations

&

Are we really going back to Bogotá, we say. Another trip, expense. Additional outflow.

Of all the doctors we've seen, there is none like Elsa, husband says. *I like that she does not say she knows. But what she says feels more certain than the claims of those who claim to know.*

I agree. No one has been so in front, so on top of situation of seizing boy.

Night seizures are bad, we say. *Even with earplugs, faint audio of boy's night seizure screams remain.*

Always, there is the Keppra, the epilepsy camp. Insurance has just confirmed second opinion for middle of May. Do we wait. Stay put. Or. Do we bring boy to Elsa, to her Cuban doctor from littoral city of Guayaquil. Discomforting stasis. To mend we decide to move.

&

As for nail-biting, I know the story begins with my father. For Father's entire life, father bit nails. Father's nails only stopped getting bit by father's mouth when father's brain lost the ability to fully control father's hands, father's mouth. Only then did his nails get long.

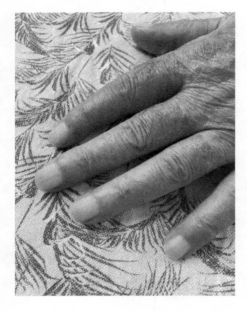

Did the part of his brain that instructs impulse to bite depart when one point five liters of blood was drained from his internally bleeding head. Did my father lose perception of anxiety requiring release via bite.

I sense anxiety still there, always there: inevitable part of even a reduced form of aware. But physical ability, coordination, mobility of bite gone. Desperation gone. If I lifted father's hand to father's mouth, would he bite. Would he appreciate the release of bite.

I bite. But not nails. I gnarl little pieces of skin that grow along the sides of nails, cuticle halfmoon wells of nails. I gnarl. Rip. Self-inflict measured bleed.

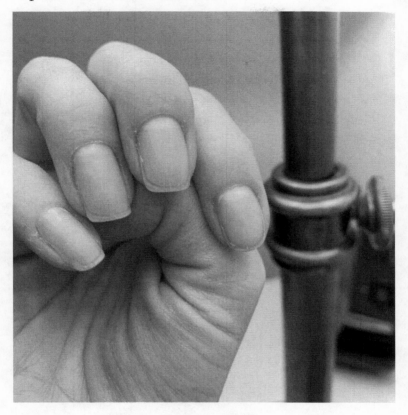

Boy bites. He bites nails hard. He even bites nails of feet. When I was little, I did too. It is my mother who sees boy biting nails of feet who tells me this.

You used to do that, she says.

Bite my nails.

That, you still do. I mean sit like that, bent, twisted, trying to get your foot in your mouth so you could bite your toenails off.

A year ago, last year, boy's teacher spoke to me after class. *We need to address boy's nail biting*, she said.

Okay, I said. *But I bite mine.* Didn't get into the whole ancestry of it. My mind inside said, let boy be. Let him access release of bite.

Grandfather, mother, boy. A clear genealogical line of bite. Genetically designed to sink teeth into selfsame hands, to sit bent, twisted, with mouth aimed at infantile feet. If it's inherited, can we call it a habit. Or is it our lot, our luck. Our providence and provenance. An outlet for congenital, cognitive angst.

&

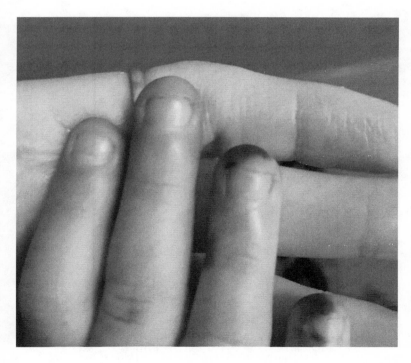

I visit friend, mom of Lionel, who is also in town for twenty-
year high school reunion fun.

I have yet to meet her baby. Baby she had after Lionel died.
Baby is beautiful. So squishy, so cute, I say.
It's been hard to get fully attached. Fully excited about things.
She's amazing.
Quiet.   More   quiet. Or is it   silence.

↳

I think sometimes that it would be easier if it happened again, she says.
Easier the second time around. Maybe it's crazy but I think about it.
It's not going to happen a second time.
Yeah. I know.
It's not.

↳

Nina's really into Willy Wonka. The Johnny Depp one. Let's talk to
her about it. It will be funny. We will laugh. Guaranteed.

&

As for compulsive vinegar ingestion, the story of trait reaches
back to my grandfather. Boy's maternal great grandfather.
Father of my father.

I remember as a child, my father pulling pickled onions
from jars at his father's house. Home-pckled onions.

I remember, too, pickled onions at the home of my father. Memories of my father excavating small round onions from jars, popping them with working hand into working mouth as if pickled onion a luscious Wonka bon-bon.

Food preserved in vinegar not my thing but pouring vinegar onto food is. So it is with boy, who will pour vinegar onto peanut butter covered toast. We keep vinegar in hard to reach drawers so boy will not decant onto food. We ration it but fail, are bad at policing, are unequipped, as parents, to prevent vinegar-drenched eggs.

Chemical composition of vinegar is this:

$$H-\overset{\displaystyle H}{\underset{\displaystyle H}{C}}-C\overset{\displaystyle O}{\underset{\displaystyle O-H}{}}$$

I look at edifice of molecule. Its covalent bonds. The scaffolding of its parts. So self-sufficient it seems. What could it possibly want from us.

&

Violet turned violet. Violet, for one, could not get away from her life.

&

As for tendency to give people nicknames so as to engage richer, swifter, interpersonal engross, I can trace trait to my father. Have no memory of older generations doing so. My grandfather was a writer: my father's father. Writing a form of nicknaming reality so perhaps that counts. Yeah, but no, probably not. Excuse my reach.

My father nicknamed all, all he serially encountered. Nicknamed several times over. Never got to nickname boy. Folds of his brain spent by the time boy was born. I am certain father does not remember name of my husband, but he remembers the nickname he gave husband.[20] Because he never was able to re-name boy, now he does not know who to ask for when he asks for boy. Father who remembers, holds on to, invented designations. Folds of his brain enfold, embrace, narrative of real world via epithet.

The first nickname boy gave was to himself. As toddler he insisted his name was Nano. Boy gives all his friends nicknames, boy's teacher, remarkably remarkable, says, *He's got one for almost all the boys. And all of them are his friends.*

Even for Messi, boy has basic nickname: Messi Man.

Months ago, boy asks me if "Messi" could be his nickname. I say no. Why not. Because it's a name that already belongs to

---

20 *El Almirante.* When I phone father, father whispers with brittle, rasping voice, says: *Cómo está el Almirante.* Father refers to my husband Nelson by way of Admiral Lord Horatio Nelson, vanquisher of Napoleonic fleet at Battle of Trafalgar. Father whose brain once contained the knowledge of an anglophile history buff. If I were to ask father for actual name of my *Almirante*, or the reason for origination of epithet, father will not always know. Sometimes he does. Other times, no.

He will not know but will also immediately recognize his inability to know. Inability that is always a surprise, this inability to know what is obvious he once knew well enough to wield. I do not ever again ask father if he knows husband's name. What does it matter anyway: the name. What matters is my father's question of husband's state. Always, always, father asks. Always, when I phone father to say hello, breakable voice remembers to ask.

someone else: to Messi. Why can't it be my nickname though, just my nickname. Well, okay, sure, I guess it could. But why don't you use "Messi Man" as your nickname. No, boy says. Why not. Because that's already Messi's nickname.

Perhaps a nickname, an espoused, self-given name, weighs more. Belongs more. Boy believes Messi Man is taken, is occupied. But Messi, just Messi, is not. Messi available for boy to adopt.

When boy picks Messi as nickname, codename, codeword, epithet, sobriquet for "seizure," his teacher, remarkably remarkable, and I say, yes. We laugh. Laugh and say, *of course*.

&

After finishing Lispector, I begin (by chance, by choice!) with Anne Carson, of the assiduously tragic, assiduously Greek. How I wish I could send Jonathan a copy of Carson's *Autobiography of Red*. It is salvation, salvation via page.

Carson unveils her story by speaking of epithet. Epithet: a nickname for nickname. She launches her story by speaking of words and names & consumption. Of how adjectives are what give names a way into, a way through, life. How adjectives order via description. How they become "the latches of being." In the selection of one specific depiction out of the infinite field of possibilities, life becomes. In the same way DNA activates proteins into traits, adjectives sketch the arches of a face. Is vs. become.

My father, the nicknamer. Boy, too, nicknames. Terms of endearment, terms of control. It's not just the conquistador, the cartographer, who seeks to name. It is the loving parent. The adoring fan. The charming, generous father I had. Once.

"Pupina": Italian for little doll. The cypher is little doll. Come what burden, what blessing may: I answer, I turn my body when the audible word of "Pupina" is said.

My father, the nicknamer. Boy, too, nicknames. Terms of endearment, terms of control. It's not just the conquistador, the cartographer, who seeks to name. It is the loving parent. The adoring fan. The charming, generous father I had.

The doctor, too, when doctor knows, names.

I only have adjectives for seizure. I do not have a name. Epilepsy names the map. Not the place. Idiopathic, disruptive, remarkable. Not enough. I want a name. Lamplight gleamed upon a name.

&

Who, in real world, will help me decipher test results of boy's DNA. If you are out there, pray tell, pray speak.

&

I speak to friend, mom of baby Anaya. I tell her of boy. She tells me of baby. Both, mid-April, seem okay.

We are waiting, she says, *for her counts to rise.*

What happens then.

Then we begin chemo, immunotherapy. Doctors haven't really been clear on when things will restart. On how. Not exactly. You know how they are. We are just waiting around for now.

Are counts still low from radiation therapy.

Yep. Anaya is still radioactive.

Wait. What. What do you mean.

I am not altogether sure what it means. What radioactive means. I can't quite wrap my brain around it all. Just that she's radioactive. I have to be careful with her pee.

Huh. Just her pee, not her poop. Or both.

Ha. Yep. Mostly her pee. But I guess all her diapers now really. We had someone from health services, or some agency like that, stop by randomly.

What. Because of her pee.

Yep. We were just throwing out her diapers with trash. The building where we are staying is not far from Trump Tower. Apparently her pee was picked up by the Secret Services. Well not her pee. The radiation from her pee. They had been hunting block by block, apartment by apartment, looking for the source. Now we have to deposit her diapers in a special bag that they pick up.

That is nuts.

It is.

It's even pretty funny. I hope you made them sweat.

Ha. Pretty sure we did.

You need to write all these stories down.

I am.

&

If DNA is keyboard of source, then mutation is what. Accidental, incidental mis-stroke of pinkie finger of source.

No.

Intentional stroke. Message evoked. Seizure, God wrote.

&

When I, designed for excessive sleep, would not wake as child, my father sang this song to wake me up—

Estas son las mañanitas
Que cantaba el Rey David
Hoy por ser día de tu santo
Te las cantamos a ti

Despierta mi bien despierta
Mira que ya amaneció
Ya los pajarillos cantan
La luna ya se metió

It is the Mexican birthday song. It is called 'Las Mañanitas': the little mornings. The small. A song sung by all the Mexican mariachi greats on YouTube and in real world. A love song. (Lovesong!) An un-sad love song because it is sung to a beloved who is there to celebrate a birthday. *El día de tu santo*: the day of your saint: the day of your birth.[21]

When I, excessive sleeper, would not wake ever on time, my father used to enter my room & sing. I remember him singing by door frame. His face a laughing face because he enjoyed singing to me while I hid under covers. I remember him call to me by one of his many nicknames for me: Aurora, Sleeping Beauty's first name. *Aurora, despierta.*

My father knew the words of many Mexican mariachi songs. He also knew the first name of Sleeping Beauty. He was a person who knew many things because of excessive books. From him comes my trait of excessive books. A trait that is not my own. Was, is, his. Our shared trait of excessive books.

———

21 Here is my translation of father's little mornings mariachi love song:

These are the mornings
Of which King David sang
And as today is your saint's day
We sing the song for you

Wake up my sweet wake up
Look the sun is risen
Already the birds are singing
And the moon has gone to bed

I do not sing Las Mañanitas to Nina Real. Even though I know the words with which to sing, even though she does not wake. I do not call her "Aurora," though she's another daughter who does not wake. I do not choose to share. I do not replicate. Do not express the trait of morning mariachi to sweet sleeping daughter who does not wake.

Why not. Why not share if sharing means that life goes on, life of father, remarkable father, lives on. Illness of father, despite.

Is the problem at hand the fact that did I not get the *Mañanitas* gene. Do I not carry the singing-to-daughter-in-morning-with-joy-gene: is it not within me, built-in. Is my lack of song not choice, but chance. Trait that did not, at random, replicate. Songless mornings a result of happenstance.

Yet—always the choice to rise above. The choice to keep the loving genius of dying father alive. As my father did, do I.

Can I. Can I activate choice, circumvent chance. Signal the difference between chance & choice. Is this difference not the same as that between song and voice.

Beyond design, beyond DNA, there is that I, this I. Hi, I. Consciousness as a dialogue between my I's.

I of excessive book, I of excessive sleep. But I, also, who observes. I who watches myself not give, for now, love song. The I who hoards Aurora. The I who stores Las Mañanitas within my brain's sole folds. But I, also, who asks in faith to be better, to be more.

It is easier to consider that if I do not reciprocate is it because some sharing gene did not replicate. It is easy to shrug. Such is life. But I know, perceive, presage it is not so. A greater inner knowingness at work.

If give of love song is choice, is decision available to me, then I believe I am designed to evolve so as to become a giver of song. Evolve to become like father past. Me, who will one day will the song of mornings forever small. I believe one morning I will choose to sing. I believe sleepy Nina Real will grow to know my father's morning daughter song.

I do. I believe. I am.

&

At the end of cruel April, on the April full moon, we find ourselves breeding lilacs out of harsh land: back again at Elsa's cloud mountain office habitat. Back again: lashing through traffic brick blocks of Bogotá's grey smog, this time to meet Cuban doctor from littoral, fluvial town of Guayaquil. Each trip, each consult, a stirring of dry tubers, a hunt for lilacs within stark land.

We arrive. Are walked in. Elsa offers tea. First time ever, in a decade of consults, Elsa offers tea. We are led, prepared. Are told to leave our phones behind, our shoes. Are taken into room lined with books in a more private part of the house. A study, Elsa's study. A gigantic German shepherd lolls in the middle of the room.

Don't talk to doctor about what boy has, Elsa says, as we sit in room's liberal, low couch. Dog slouches over to us. Boy recoils. Despite, dog is slow. *He has arthritis,* Elsa says. *I'll take him out and be right back*. Elsa steps out with dog and leaves us in room, but we are not alone.

Cuban doctor sits behind a desk. What surprises me is his shape. Not lean like all my other witch doctors, whose bodies reflect years of conscious food ingestion. But round. Uncle round. Priest plump. Casual waist of casual ingest. Cuban doctor is not witch doctor I sense.

Doctor performs his own scan: wires attach to boy's head as before, as in EEG. Boy is sad. He is visibly, audibly sad. On a cot he must lie flat. Outside in Elsa's driveway, he saw space and a soccer ball. *When we are done, you can play*, Elsa says.

After forty minutes, doctor is done. He asks us to sit by his side. Hands us report printed by assistant with printer set up in dark corner of room. Elsa leads boy out to play.

Do you have something to write with, doctor says.

No. We left all our things at entry of house.

Here. Take this pen. Take this paper. Write down what I am about to say.

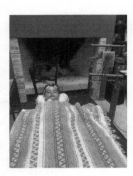

&

&

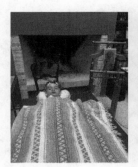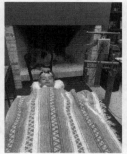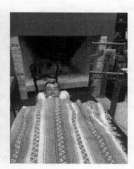

There are different types of brain waves. Mostly we have delta, theta, alpha. Are you writing this down.

I am not. I begin to write, to take, down: delta, theta, alpha.

Delta are the waves that correspond to our first years, to when we are babies. The waves that generate automatic functioning. Crying, eating, sleeping. Theta are the waves that correspond to the next stage. To language and walking, to balance. Then we have alpha. Alpha corresponds to intellectual development. Between delta, theta and alpha are ninety percent of the brain's waves. Then we have some ten percent in beta. Brain waves transition from one type to the other from birth up until we turn six or seven. When they don't transition correctly, seizures can emerge. I see from scan that boy is having seizures. Seizures result from excessive energy in delta. Brain has electrical discharges because brain is not operating at the correct voltage, correct frequency. Brain needs to release excessive electricity. Okay.

Okay.

Boy has a process of dis-maturation. His waves are not maturing correctly. Write that down. Process. Of. Dis-maturation. What does boy have.

Doctor is silent. We are silent.

What does boy have.

A process of dis-maturation.

Write that down. Okay.

Okay.

What are the brain waves. The names.

We are silent.

Are you paying attention.

Yes, we say. *Delta and beta,* husband says.

No. Write what I say. Delta. Theta. Alpha. Problem of boy is in Theta. Also Delta. Also, look at this. This red area you see in this map, here, is a focus of aggression. Is he impulsive, aggressive at times. Bad temper.

Yes. Very much so.

This is not surprising. Most Colombians I've scanned have it.

We laugh. Doctor does not.

It's true, Elsa says. *It's completely true. Most of the patients we've scanned here have it.*

We stop laughing. It's not funny. It is true.

Boy also has a focus of addiction. Is he addictive in general. Has a harder time than you think normal of letting go. Video games. Food. Things like that.

Yes. Very much so. He is hyper-focused. Single-minded. Hyper-active as well.

Okay. Well the hyper-activity is also explained by what I see here. He cannot help it. No use fighting too much with him. He has over-active frequencies of brain. This other area in red here means boy has bad perception of reality. He sees things worse than they are. Does he seem sad sometimes, takes things the wrong way. Depressive. In a way that seems excessive. And can last for days.

*He does. His moods come and go. But when they come, they do last
for days. It's tough to handle him then. What do you think of medication.
Doctors prescribed Keppra. Would the Keppra help.*

Cuban doctor calls out across room to assistant who printed
scan for us.

*Damaris. Damaris, what do you give a kid if you want to poison
him.*

Keppra, Damaris says.

*If you want to poison boy give boy Keppra. Keppra is toxic. Okay.
Okay. So what do you recommend.*

*Listen. I don't need new patients. I have more than I need. But I can
help boy. You can schedule with my center & come. I can regulate his frequencies. Help his theta make the correct switch over to alpha. Treatment
takes about a month. I'll treat boy in Guayaquil.*

&

Elsa takes us back to her regular office after consult with Cuban
doctor is done. She looks at us, expectant.

*Listen, doctor can be tough, but his treatment works. I've seen
incredible things happen at his center. The kids I've sent come back transformed. Perhaps boy does not have terrible form of epilepsy but no doubt
there are behavioral issues attached to his epilepsy. You could save yourself
ten years of strife by going to Guayaquil once. Maybe twice.*

We are quiet. Silent.

*Listen, doctor will find fault with anyone he scans. We all have some-
thing wrong with us. Our faults are our story: what we came to this life
to learn, to overcome. I know the doctor says things in a difficult way.
But his treatment corrects harmful tendencies. It's not that the treatment
changes the person, it's just that it can help correct impulsive, aggressive
behaviors that are not helpful. Not to mention eliminate seizure activity*

*in the brain. Seizures are dangerous. It is not something we want the boy
to live with. It is not through seizure that any of us want story of his life
to evolve.*

We are silent. Quiet.

*Listen, let me take a look at boy quickly. Haven't seen him in a
month. You've kept the diet up, right. No dairy, no sugar, no gluten.
The vitamins, the belladonna.*

Yes. We have.

Seizing still, but only night, right.

*Yes. Only at night. Stronger seizures, longer seizures. But only at
night.*

Elsa inspects boy. We watch. Colored filters placed along boy's
center line. Elsa's hands that move, convene, convoke. Summon,
invoke. Pause atop head, appear to draw, disperse, disband. We are
quiet but not silent. We are reticence. Exhaustion. Reserve.

*His fields are better. Seems your hard work, the changes in diet,
supplements, may be paying off. Continue to wait on the medication.
Let's stay away from Keppra. You heard what doctor said. But, I'm glad
you are going to get a second opinion. Make sure to ask them to recommend other seizure medications. When they give you medication names,
send them to me. There are better ones out there. If situation changes,
we want to be ready to respond.*

&

Tell me a story, boy says. *But don't tell me a story of your dad or mom
and then me being born. Just a normal story.*

You don't like the stories of when you were born.

*Yes. But you always tell me those. Tell me another one. Like a
normal story.*

I pause. Panic. It is so hard for me to tell stories unprepared. The ones that come are always my own. My family's. Sad stories not fit for boy. Or. Story of boy right now. I am consumed by story of unwell boy. Not a normal story. Not an only happy story. But an only story. The story of the boy who shook.

&

It's all of it, Eli says, while her hands, her *manitas,* lie static on boy. *All you are doing. All of it. Combined. All of it together seems to be working. Boy is better. What did Elsa say.*

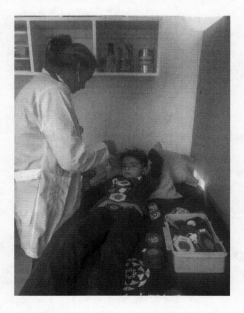

To be prepared. To ask for another seizure medication. To consider Ecuador. But yes, that boy seems better, stronger.

Yes, you need to be prepared. When it's time to medicate, it's time to medicate. I've heard Ecuador is rough, difficult. Not fun. But that it works. It's worked very well for some people. Think about it. Meanwhile

*let's continue to watch boy. This is all still so new. You have to remember:
it's only been two months. How is his digestion. I continue to feel that
part of boy's body off.*

It's not great. Never has been great.

I'll give you some drops to help him cleanse. Some Spascupreel.

What's that.

*Homeopathy for muscle seizures. Helps relax them. Replenish them.
His seem spent. You all seem spent, but better, as well.*

What do you mean.

*Boy has united all of you around him. You and husband work so
much. Have worked so much. Look at you all here. Lie down. I want to
work on you.*

What about boy. He won't just wait.

Let him play on your phone. He will be fine.

&

At airport waiting to board flight back home, away from mountain orb, the traffic fog blocks of Bogotá, in line for good coffee,
with boy beside, boy asks for Gatorade, which I will, of course,
not buy. *No, you know it's no,* I say. *But Mimi,* boy says, smiles.
But Mimi. I turn to ignore, to order my coffee and water for
boy. But before I speak: I see boy lean back into refrigerated
vending aisle: lean back & laugh.

It's happening. Boy's day seizures are back. Back to tell us all.
O, they shall tell us all.

&

I read 'Prufrock' for the first time in high school English class.
Our desks arranged into an angular U. One *Norton Anthology of*

Poetry open on each rectangular desk[22]. My desk on the right line of the rectangular U. My location engrained as memory by the folds of my electrical brain.

We do not read Prufrock in high school English class. We read Donne, John Donne. Poet of the passionate, metaphysical, near-Enlightened God. I am done with Donne. I am in high school: I am bored with God. Bored with Church and how Church becomes all the history we are taught to learn, history determined by alignment with or opposition to, not human Christ, but sovereign Church. Church of royal, papal, paper God. Spanish conquests, Protestant claims. Virginity as holy cloak.

In *Norton*, I read ahead, bored in class, to the future, to my century. To a moment I consider beyond God. To grammar I use. I find him there. At the beginning of poems anthologized under Twentieth Century, at the dawn, the impulsive pre-war start to a century my high school self considers beyond the confines of history's God.

Hola, Prufrock.

My poem gene, of course, is already inside. Dormant, but inside. Inside, within skin. My poetry DNA replicated, created at birth. Prufrock is modest, assertive, polite: of course, he says *Hi* back.

Hola, Ana. Hola, poem gene inside Ana.

I read in disbelief that becomes belief. I read beyond schedule, beyond confines of English class. I read and stop: read and repeat. Over and over & over again. Prufrock becomes belief. Prufrock is spark: electrical synapse leap who introduces me to I.

O, God. Batter, he does, my human heart.

———

22 (each to each!)

8

On May 6, 2019, I have the following real-world conversation with six-year-old boy from the span of approximately 8:15 pm to 8:40 pm, the time at which I leave him to write down what he said for fear of forgetting. But, already, when I sit to write, I forget half.

When is the instant of forget. I thought I had it. Had it all. But not all of it will make it here. Here, where I sit to write is here where I sit to forget. At least, not all is gone. Here is what I remember, what I write, & so, keep—

I ask boy, *do you feel anything or think anything about your seizures.*

It is a question I have been asking boy frequently to see if boy needs outlet to speak about what is happening. If he is internalizing. External happening internalized as intense emotional trauma that will be trouble, oh, how much trouble. Later on.

No, he says.

I tell boy Miss Lara's mother used to have seizures. Miss Lara is boy's teaching assistant.

How do you know.

Miss Lara told me. We can ask her about it tomorrow if you want.

How did her mom get seizures.

Because sometimes people get seizures. It's a thing that happens. It's not good or bad. It just happens. Do you like that you get seizures.

No.

Why. What don't you like about them.

No one else has them.

Do they make you feel different.

Yes. Because when I am playing soccer at school I need to stop.

But I thought you weren't having seizures at school. Do you get them during soccer practice after school.

Yes. No. Never during soccer practice. Only during recess. When I play soccer at recess. And it makes me have to stop playing. Because I need to sit down. And maybe I miss a shot.

I am quiet. I know boy is thinking what I am thinking. That every day after school I ask boy about seizures & he says none. I feel boy realize he has not told me about dozens, hundreds of small seizures he's had at school, elsewhere. Moments of *it's happening* but boy did not remember, did not keep, so, could not think to say.

Boy says, *I don't know why I don't remember. I only make room for good memories in my brain. I only have a few sad ones.*

What sad ones.

The tragic Spanish Civil War.

What. Why. Where did you hear about that.

Because it was so bad. I want to tell people about it. So, I remember it.

I am quiet. I remember. I know where boy learned about the tragic Spanish Civil War: a documentary boy watches called *Barça Dreams*, about the history of Barcelona's soccer team, the team where Messi, his Messi, plays.

I remember that and things about science.

But science is neither good nor bad. It's not sad. It just is. Do you think science is sad.

No. Science is not sad. But I like to keep science facts. Like when I told my class that gold, silver and uranium come from nebulae.

Being different is like science, it's not a good or bad thing, I say to boy. *It's just a thing that is.*

x/y

Still in Bogotá, the day after Cuban doctor scans brain of boy, husband wakes and says:

> *You will not believe what I am about to say.*
> *Ha. Okay. What.*
> *I feel like I am going to fall.*
> *What.*
> *It started when we got here, and I thought it was the altitude at first. That or the lack of sleep. But it's not. It's gotten worse. I don't think I can get up.*
> *What do you mean.*
> *I don't think I can get up from bed.*
> *Really.*
> *Really.*
> *Do you think we need to go to hospital.*
> *Not yet. Let's wait. Maybe it will go. Away.*
> *Okay.*

x/y

Soon it is May. April is not May. May will be better is a thing that, at the close of April, we will and say.

x/y

Boy's slight day seizure at Bogotá's airport, headed home to Miami, presages many more.

> Convulsions. *Convulsiones.*
> Episodes. *Episodios.*

One on plane. Another on ride home. A stronger, longer one in bed, right before brain, before body, drops into sleep. Yes. The right-before-sleep-seizure, old foe, is back again.

I call husband, who stayed behind in Bogotá.

I counted three. Since airport. Three.

Strong.

No. Well, the before sleep one was stronger but not terrible terrible. The usual. Like before.

Are you giving anything new.

No. Well, Eli's homeopathic antispasmodic. I mean. Nothing. Although am going to stop that of course.

Yes. Stop it for sure.

Okay.

Okay. Let's wait. Maybe he's tired from the trip. Maybe the altitude. Maybe day seizures will go back away.

Okay.

x/y

Incidentally, there is always a nun to be spotted inside the airport of the mountain orb of Bogotá. Go ahead, play spot-the-nun when next or ever you fly into or out of the plateau climb of Bogotá.

x/y

Husband's feeling of falling does not go away. In Bogotá, that day, that morning, husband cannot get out of bed.

Okay, he says.

Okay you are better.

No. Okay let's go to hospital.

Okay. Let's go to the one we went to when my dad got sick.

Yes, okay.

x/y

When I need music for literary purposes, I often start with *'Bird on a Wire'* by Leonard Cohen.

Is this what Ariana Reines heard when she wrote the words I was listening to Bob Dylan and Leonard/Cohen in order to think about/you for literary purposes. A song played so many times. Overplayed. Yet. It is a line I refuse to think of as saturated, old, overdone, overdid. As in mind-numbing: trite, not again: bored.[23]

Song continues to provoke feeling of literary. Feeling of it is possible to write a book that is my life but somehow on paper and it will make sense on paper and be both solid and fragile more fragile than off paper because undeniable and exposed. Suddenly unhidden reality of hidden familiar world.

Summarized: the feeling of I have tried in my way to be free is the feeling of sit & try to write a book.

x/y

Are you sure you want to come. You don't need to.

Of course I'll come. Kids are happy here with abuelos. Plus, it'll be a good time for me to read. Let's just pack a bag. We can leave it in car.

Really. A bag.

I'll pack it quickly.

We get to hospital and nothing is quick about hospital. Husband tells them he has feeling he is going to fall. Hands flat on counter. Has to hold on to stand.

We find place to sit. An empty plastic bench: here we will find no empty Turkish seats.

I do not read. I watch Colombian morning shows on waiting

___

23 See start of Chapter 6 for more on overdid.

room TV. It feels like a break. To sit and watch bad somehow foreign somehow domestic TV. All morning shows are the same morning show. The same morning. The same show. The same wait. For day to consume us until we feel awake.

You want a coffee, I say.

Sure.

We sit & sip & wait. *Café con leche* not mark but liquid balm within our cupped hands.

x/y

Compulsive vinegar consumption, nail biting, nicknaming. Cravings, hungers, physical, psychological coveting that tie me to boy, me to father, my father to boy: tie us three.

A synonym for compulsive is neurotic. Neurotic as in fixated, as in single-minded. Us three of a single genetic mind, a single, slowly evolving, manifestation of synoptic idiosyncrasy, electrical eccentricity. The same fabric cut.

Ancestral foibles regurgitated, partially digested, mildly elevated. The same fabric chopped. By choice, by chance, by force, by happenstance. Fabric, despite its patterns, despite its current edits and iterations, that remains cloth.

So slowly. So slowly, we evolve.

I bite the skin from my cuticles as I write. The angst of unknowing feels the same as the angst of sensing why.

x/y

"Nelson David" is called. We stand.

You can walk okay.

Yes. Fine. I feel better actually. It's gone down.

Colombian hospital coffee. Good every time.

x/y

A few synonyms for "aura" as included, in this specific order, by Microsoft® Word for Mac Version 16.26:

air (n.)
atmosphere
feeling
impression
sensation
characteristic
quality
appearance
force
glow

"Liminal" is not word included as term.

x/y

Should I go in with him.
   No, please wait here.
   The young doctor points toward the smaller interior waiting room to which she has led us.
   I wait, sit. No coffee. No TV. I do not pull out book to read. I do nothing and something with the lit electromagnetic screen that is my phone.

x/y

I cannot get this quote by Alain Badiou out of brain, out of mind. A quote I read in Ariana Reines' book *Mercury*—
   "Because an event is pure rapture, an event disappears immediately: it does not exist objectively but only by appearing and disappearing."

I think of phrase in relation to boy's events. Boy's episodes. Boy's Messi raptures. Boy's enrapture for and with soccer superstar Lionel Messi. Lifespan of baby Lionel. What is this world that is real. This world of incident. Is it all event. All rapture. Watch it disappear.

x/y

Husband emerges with young doctor. She points my way. Husband sits next to me.

What happened. Are you okay. What did she say.

I have vertigo. She laid me down and moved my head. I felt like I would fall into the bed. But she says what she did will make me feel better soon.

Vertigo.

Yes. Vertigo.

Did she say why.

I told her about boy. She says vertigo is usually stress-related. So.

Oh. Now what.

I'm getting discharged. She is filing all the paperwork. Getting medicine they prescribed. You'll never guess what.

What.

Dramamine.

x/y

We are discharged: head to restaurant we saw on way to ER.

What do you think of Cuban doctor, I say when we sit.

He seems like a scientist. Very thorough. Reading was impressive. He nailed boy. Whatever it is he knows, he definitely knows. I have no doubt he could help us.

Yes.

It's far though. And expensive. And long. I don't know about that trip. I'm not sure.

I know, I say. It's such a difficult trip. Boy seems to be better.

Yes. He does.

Is that Sting.

What.

The music. Is that Sting.

Wait. It is. Never heard this one before.

Me neither. Let me Shazzam it. It's a song called 'Sad Trombone.' *By Sting and Shaggy.*

It's good. Save it.

Guess you're better, I say.

Must be the Dramamine.

x/y

Boy is not better.

Back in Miami: his seizures of day of night so bad we lose count. Ten fifteen twenty per twenty-four-hour planetary swirl.

Seismic volcanic meteoric yet persistently organic micro-scopic   trip.

x/y

My husband's chiropractor: another Cuban doctor, but from Miami. A man whose name—no joke—is Dr. Bravo. The man, the doctor, who cured husband's broken sacrum some ten years ago. Husband, recovered from vertigo, now cannot move neck. Takes boy with him to fix his neck. Chiropractor is witch doctor. One we forgot to consult.

It is the week of seizure spike. Two weeks before second opinion. Time of surrender. We surrender here before this thing we have. Epilepsy is event. And event is all we are.

Bring boy tomorrow, Dr. Bravo says. *Bring him at the end of the day. I will need some time with him. But I have seen this before. Several times, I have seen this occur. It is something that, with time, I can cure. Traémelo mañana.*

Traémelo. Traémelo. Traémelo.

x/y

In a writing class, I share the first chapter of this book of seizure of boy. In class, I read other works. One is written in the format of boy's genetic test results. I ask its writer why.

My boyfriend runs the genetic lab at Florida International University, he says. *So even though his work is basically illegible to me, I thought the format interesting, so I borrowed it.*

I got genetic results back from test we ran on boy. Do you think I could ask your boyfriend to coffee and he can help me sift through boy's results. Please, do you think.

Absolutely. He's done it for friends before. I'd like to come, too. Write me and we will speak.[24]

x/y

Whereas before boy insisted on sleeping with me, with husband

---

24 The Gospel of Matthew, Chapter 7, Verses 7-8, KJV:

7. Ask, and it shall be given you; seek, and ye shall find; knock, and it shall be opened unto you:
8. For every one that asketh receiveth; and he that seeketh findeth; and to him that knocketh it shall be opened.

and me. We speak to him and say: *we, mommy, daddy, we need sleep. At night, you don't realize, but you are having seizures, episodes. They wake mommy and daddy up and we cannot sleep. We need to sleep. You have to sleep in your bed in your own room. So that we can sleep.*

Okay.

You understand.

Yes.

We take boy to his bed in his room. No fight. No argument. No negotiating. Surrender. Acquiescence. Concession.

Mimi, but can we still snuggle puff until I fall asleep.

Of course, baby.

Once I return to my room husband asks—

Did he say anything else.

No.

Did you.

No, I just stayed with him until he fell asleep. He understood.

Husband is quiet. Room is quiet. House is quiet. Immaculate quiet. Quiet as the Keppra perched atop our kitchen shelf.

x/y

(am I not here with you, I, who am your mother)

x/y

On May 7, 2019, boy goes to cousin's house. To play. We are weary of playdates but always so positive. Okay, we say. Go play. While there, boy falls off counter chair. The seizure caught on video. From first idiopathic giggle to final fall, a span of thirty-six seconds. No day seizure has lasted this long before.

My brother sent me the video, husband says. *Are you sure you want to see it.*

Yes.
You don't have to.
I want to see it.
It's going to make you cry. I cried.
Lo quiero ver.
Okay.

We enter still real new world: confinement of perpetual terror realm. The countdown begins. One week, seven days, one hundred and sixty-eight hours, until the day when we wake, and it's second opinion time.

x/y

There is always worse. *To husband,* I say. Go online, go. There is always worse. We need to stay positive and grateful.

But what I think, what I will to say, no longer works: there is nothing left to rationalize, to reconsider, to dip in big good coffee mug. Not when it's fifteen or more seizures per day. Not when the sound of boy drop is caught on real world digital videotape.

New adjectives, epithets, emerge: shattering, disruptive, wounding, life-threatening. We send video to our Colombian witch doctors. To all.

Elsa, as always, though the busiest, is first to call. *Increase belladonna to three times per day, add another homeopathic medicine called silicea, five globules four times per day, no video games, absolutely no sugar. But know, this is just a band aid until you go get your second opinion. Your goal when you go is to come back with the right medication for boy.*

It is time, she says, *to medicate.*

x/y

Chiropractor no longer just fixes backs: Dr. Bravo fixes all: disease of ingredients of life.

You will not know if it was me or everything else you did that healed boy, Dr. Bravo says. *But it will be me. I don't say it like I am so great. Believe me. But it will simply be me. I have seen a lot of this. A lot of what boy has. What he has is going around a lot lately. Because of all the electronics in our life. I healed a girl no medication, not even surgery, could heal. Bad cases. Worse than yours. Much worse.*

I need to show you video of bad seizure boy just had, I say, *one that made boy fall.*

I don't need to see it. I can imagine it. Don't worry, what I am doing will make it stop.

Aura of doctor, which I am able to observe at length during this, boy's second two-hour consult, is completely, remarkably yellow. Yellow as yellow lamplight.

While Dr. Bravo works, I delve web of internet to find meaning of yellow aura: emerging psychic, awakening, positive about new ideas.

Before, I would not have been able to do this, doctor says. *I am much better at reading the body than I was before. I now have my own technique. My own language. I can connect to boy's body, to another's body, via movement of my hands.*

I attempt to be positive about new ideas. But boy is restless. Even though beloved cousin Sebastian is with us this time. Boy asks, *Mimi can we watch iPad.* I look at doctor.

Actually, it's okay. They can watch it. Our bodies are supposed to be able to eliminate electromagnetic contamination, which is everywhere these days. But boy's body is compromised, debilitated. Night seizures and lack of sleep don't help. His sleep quality is at three percent. Of course, he has a predisposition to seizures. But there is more here. Don't worry. I am working on it as we speak.

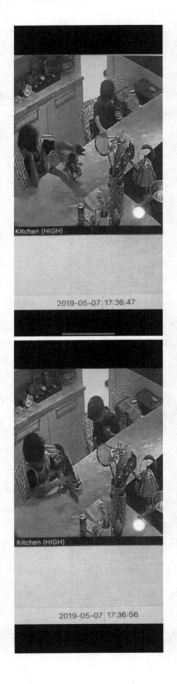
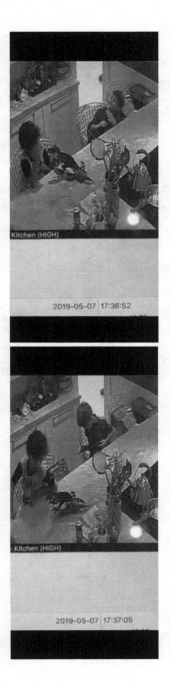

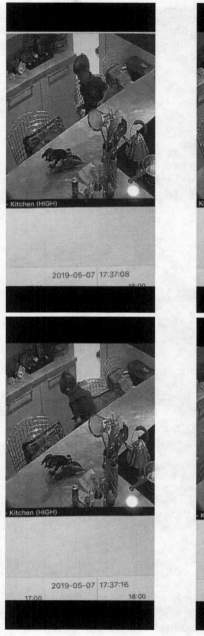

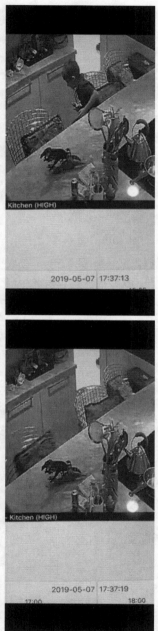

Doctor moves own hands within each other. He tells me he is asking a series of questions about boy. The way hands move are response. Rigidity, flexibility of muscles in his own hands speak, bare what boy lacks, reveal what boy overly, overtly has. Similar to what Dr. Carmona, to what Elsa, to what Eli, to what Sergio, to what Lucy, have done. Each witch with a specific language of hands.

Do you believe in God, I say. With my other witch doctors, faith, belief, not question but fact. Their faith announced to entire real world. But with Dr. Bravo, I am unsure.

I do. But, I didn't before.

Before what.

Before I started being able to work like this with my hands.

What do you mean.

The answers I get come from somewhere that is not me. Somewhere that is higher than me, doctor shrugs, continues to speak, as if to no one, in that certain, simple way he speaks.

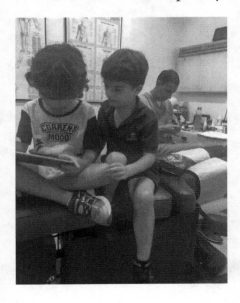

Like how I can tell you boy has a predisposition to seizure, Dr. Bravo says, *and his system is weakened. Weakened, but recovering. He lost ability to remove build-up of electromagnetic toxicity. Also. He has entities attached, four of them. Dark energies. I don't usually tell my patients this. It freaks them out. But it happens all the time. Nothing to be afraid of. Just something to remove. Something to purge.*

I pause, then say, *I've had an entity before. At least one. It was removed. I felt it on me. I didn't know what it was, but I knew something was up. Something foreign to me, affecting me. I called a medium who lives in Monterey. She discovered it when she sensed its shadow rim move. She removed it over the phone. Burped, as she worked. I broke out into heavy cold sweat. I almost puked. I could barely drive myself to a meeting an hour after we hung up.*

Boy's is very hard to remove, doctor says. *It's gotten comfortable. But I got a lot done today. Bring him back next week. I should be done then.*

Can you work over the phone.

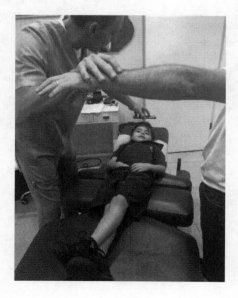

Yes.

We leave for our second opinion next week. Can we do it from there.

Yes. Dr. Bravo pauses, then says, *they are going to tell you to medicate.*

Yes.

If you medicate, you'll never know what healed boy. And you'll be afraid to let go of the medication.

I am quiet. A quiet longer than pause.

Heal. Cure. Know. These words, these things. Their combination of. For the first time, I do not care to name the terms I fail to know.

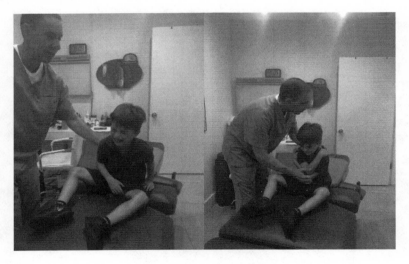

x/y

Dark energy is not to be confused with cosmological dark energy, the energy propelling the universe apart.

Cosmological dark energy is already so confusing. The universe is expanding. Expanding at an acceleration increasing at a rate faster than it should.

It was hard for scientists to believe in accelerated universal expansion, acceleration & expansion despite gravity's pull. A shift in belief had to occur to accommodate observed behaviors of the real world.

In 2008, reporter Dennis Overbye wrote in *The New York Times*—[25]

"Although cosmologists have adopted a cute name, dark energy, for whatever is driving this apparently antigravitational behavior on the part of the universe, nobody claims to understand why it is happening, or its implications for the future of the universe and of the life within it, despite thousands of learned papers, scores of conferences and millions of dollars' worth of telescope time. It has led some cosmologists to the verge of abandoning their fondest dream: a theory that can account for the universe and everything about it in a single breath."

Scientists can be funny, sometimes, when they realize they do not know—

"When astronomers and physicists gathered at the Space Telescope Science Institute recently to take stock of the revolution, their despair of getting to the bottom of the dark energy mystery anytime soon, if ever, was palpable, even as they anticipate a flood of new data from the sky in coming years. When it came time for one physicist to discuss new ideas about dark energy, he showed a blank screen."

Blank because we do not know enough to say. Not even now, eleven years after article above was written, do we know much more.

---

25 https://www.nytimes.com/2008/06/03/science/03dark.html

In 2019, reporter Dennis Overbye writes in *The New York Times*—[26]

"If dark energy remains constant, everything outside our galaxy eventually will be moving away from us faster than the speed of light, and will no longer be visible. The universe will become lifeless and utterly dark. But if dark energy is temporary — if one day it switches off — cosmologists and metaphysicians can all go back to contemplating a sensible tomorrow."

I snort when I read this. For I, maternal metaphysician, domestic cosmologist—I, too, contemplate a sensible tomorrow. One in which boy's dark energy, his accelerated deterioration, is temporary. Switched off by the work of human hands and the grace of that which fills empty space.

But, back to the heavens. The slices of universal substance look like this—

Real world

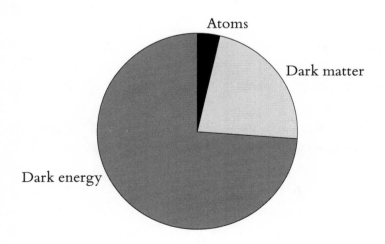

---

26 https://www.nytimes.com/2019/02/25/science/cosmos-hub-
ble-dark-energy.html

Infinite, it seems, are the ways the material universe is meant to be yanked apart. What looks empty really is not. The vacuum, its order, is not dark. It is smart. Somehow creation of planet-home occurred.

Here we are: lit like lamplight, celestial mixture of chance and choice. Self-aware manifestation of atomic form. At once the thing & its combination of.

x/y

He needs to stay on the ground, I say to director of boy's school. *Other than that, he should be fine. We leave in a few days for a week to see another doctor. Hopefully we'll come back with some answers.*

I agree. He should be fine. Plus, Miss Lara will keep her eye on him the whole time.

Absolutely, Miss Lara says.

How'd the kids in class react this morning when you told them, I say.

They were great. I told them they needed to keep an eye on boy and if he ever started acting funny to let a teacher know immediately. Some of them had noticed it, I think. They did not seem surprised. They will help me keep him safe.

I asked boy if he wanted to be there when you spoke. But he was really upset about it. Very embarrassed. That's why we came in late.

No worries. I told the kids that it was something private. They all really got it. You should have seen them. They have his back.

x/y

Some time following boy's counter stool fall, I reread collection of poems by poet Charles Simic. A collection I could not remember reading but soon realize the words had been inside my head before. Notes made by my own physical hands inside pages of book.

I read, reread, these lines—

I believe in the soul; so far
It hasn't made much difference.

I understand something about poem, finally. Poem is simply an idea, an idea & the gut of getting it down on paper. The gut of capture. Seizing time to capture event.

From there—from gut, from capture—good poem is function of practice. Patient practice, however, is also from and of the gut. It is surmounting fear. Surmounting the fear of wasted time writing and rewriting poem. Next comes faith. Here, body is again required. Faith that poem in hands is good. No longer fear of capture, but belief of matter. There is a difference. The difference of gut vs. mind.

It takes so long to understand simple things.[27] For example: one life. For example: one gut, one mind. Will this life, this gut, this mind, be poem. Will I seize time. Will I usurp or be usurped. Will I have enough to say.

O, God. O, will. O, say.

x/y

You need to understand this is evolution in action.
    Seizures, I say.
    No. Mutations.
    Right.
We, husband and I, are sitting at coffee shop with friend from writing class and his boyfriend, who runs genetic lab at university I attend.
    Let me first explain what's on the page. Boy has two mutations.

---

27 So slowly, so slowly, we evolve.

You'll see on report they are both classified as VOUS. This means Variants of Unknown Significance. This means we don't have a freaking clue what this means. Keep in mind, unknown does not mean bad. Both are heterozygous. Do you know what that means.

The way we move our heads says *no.*

We all have two copies of each gene in our body, one copy from each parent. In boy's case, for these two genes with mutations on them, each copy of the gene is different. That's good because mutation is only on one copy. One of the two. We can assume he has one normal copy and one mutated copy.

Like a spare.

Kind of, yes. There shouldn't be a complete loss of function. We just don't know. Not for sure.

Okay.

One of the mutations is AD the other AR. One is autosomal domi- nant and the other is autosomal recessive. Do you understand what this means.

The way our faces look says *no.*

We each have twenty-three pairs of chromosomes. Of the twenty- three, one pair are the sex chromosomes: X/Y. The other twenty-two pairs are the autosomes. He's got mutations on genes that are not sex genes. We tend to think of autosomal dominance as the result of inheri- tance, but it can also happen due to mutation. Just one autosomal dom- inant copy is enough for the underlying trait or disorder or whatever to express. With an autosomal recessive trait, you need two recessive copies for expression.

Our faces are flat: they say *go on.*

Your kids are not exactly half of you. Not quite. When sperm & egg combine random mutations can occur. Also, alleles from mom and dad recombine. All this increases genetic diversity and drives evolution.

Mistakes can also happen. You probably learned about Mendel in high school. He's the guy we call the "Father of Genetics." The guy that did all that famous work on the pea plant. His laws basically say that recombination is mutation.[28]

What's an allele.

It's just a kind of a gene. A type. So, for example, there are genes for eye color. And we say there is an allele for blue eyes, an allele for brown eyes, and so on. We each have two alleles for each gene, two variants of each gene, although, of course, we could have two alleles that are the same. During reproduction all four alleles, two from mom and two from dad, recombine. Are you with me.

The way our mouths move says, tentatively, *yes.*

Alleles, genes determine what proteins our bodies make. There's a total of twenty amino acids. These are strung together into different proteins. Proteins then combine to become genes. And genes then determine what our body builds and does. So, for example, here, in boy's first mutation, there is an amino acid change at position 50 of the CHRNA2 *gene. Proline is changed to leucine. That's what the p.P50L on the genetic test means.*

What are these changes measured against. How do we know what's supposed to be.

We have a standard for normal. Based on lots of past genetic tests performed. Obviously, normal is a work in progress. The first mutation appears to be on a gene that codes for ions. Sort of the way our bodies conduct electricity. The second mutation, the autosomal recessive one, is related to fat production. See where it says p.R97C. This means there is a change from arginine to cysteine at position 97 of the gene.

We are quiet. Our oval faces say *scared.*

---

28 Not the thing, but the (re)combination of.

Okay, so what I am trying to explain is that in boy's case, in both mutations, full proteins are made. Just one amino acid is switched. Like in a car, if you change a part of the car, the car will run differently. But it can still run. These changes appear to be fully viable. Fully compatible with life. These mutations are changes that are simply a part of who boy is. In the first one, the one related to ions, perhaps boy is overactive. Maybe this mutation translates to something like a hyperactive nervous system.

Absolutely. He has so much energy. Too much. Mentally & physically.

In the second one, the one related to fat production, it's probably safe to say that boy needs to eat differently. He may just need a ton of butter. Bacon & butter. Buckets of lard. Although since this one is recessive it may not manifest.

Ha. He is so thin. Small in every way for his age.

So again. This is all part of evolution. Part of who boy, genetically, is. What have doctors said.

To be honest, we didn't understand a word our doctor here said. We are leaving in a few days to get a second opinion. Our doctor here never explained, never even mentioned anything like what you just said. It was as if he didn't think we could handle the information or like it wasn't worth his time. He seemed reluctant to even give us a copy of these results.

It's nuts. I don't get why doctors in Miami are so paternalistic. It's good you are getting a second opinion.

We've been doing a lot of alternative medicine as well. Making changes in diet, acupuncture, energy work. Things like that.

Listen, none of that can hurt. But I'd say boy likely has an underlying proclivity for seizures. A predisposition. You've heard of epigenetics though.

Yes. Some.

Epigenetics basically refers to things that control expression of certain genes but do not actually change our genetic makeup. Diet, sleep habits, stuff like that can definitely alter how our genetics translate into visible life. Honestly, the blunt truth is that there is so much we still don't know. In terms of sleep, for example, scientists still don't fully understand why animals need sleep.

What do you mean.

Evolutionarily, it makes no sense. Sleep is a huge risk. Plants don't sleep. They have rhythms but that's not quite sleep. It's possible sleep is related to memory. That at night the brain cuts down the number of active synapses to filter out what it will keep from all that happened in your day. You don't remember every single moment, yet you remember some.

Ha. That's wild.

It is. You mentioned boy's seizures seem to come from his right frontal lobe. That's the most plastic part of the brain. It won't finish developing until he is twenty-five. He may grow out of this. Then again, he may not. But there are great medications out there for epilepsy. I am sure you will find a way to live with what he has.

x/y

A pictorial/textual rendition of material conversation with geneticist and of how it atmospherically feels—

Genetics vs. Epigenetics:

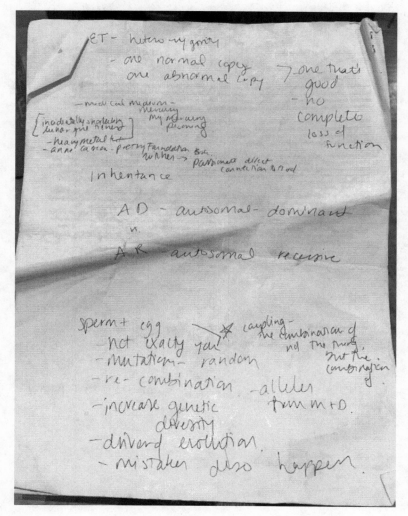

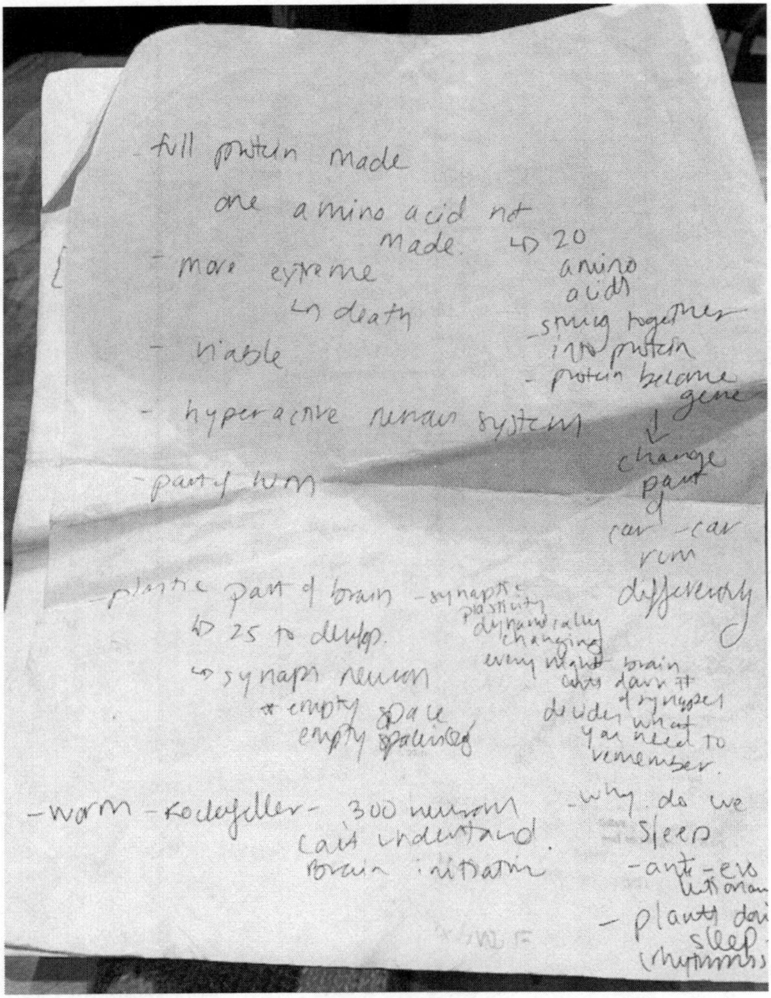
- full protein made
one amino acid not made.
20 amino acids string together into protein
- protein became gene
- more extreme
death
- viable
- hyperactive
system
change part of car - car run differently
- plastic part of brain - synaptic plasticity
25 to develop.
dynamically changing
every night brain
synapse neuron
empty space
decides what you need to remember.
- worm - rockefeller - 300 neurons
can't understand brain initiation
- why do we sleep
- plants do sleep

(Notes, over coffee, over & over, relived, reread.)

- coding region = makes the protein
    basically the same
        btwn ppl + animals

- epigenetics vs. epigenetics =
        ↓   ↓
    turns that   - the changes
    control   in DNA.
    expression   - ch 8 - HET
    but does   progressive illness
    not   - genetically designed
    change   to many feet

- Mendels law
    (recombination is the)
            mutation

- women =
    mosaics
    XX - are inactivated

x/y

We come home from chat with geneticist and boy has built a fort with cushions of couch. Pillows, blankets, throws. Within fort boy includes his vitamins. His water. All the substances he is inserting.

Is this who boy thinks he is. A being usurped. Seizure, not part of him, but the whole. And is it us, husband and me, his parents, who keep him this way. Who keep him seizing, keep him usurped.

Predisposition, sure. Dark energy, parasites, bad diet, bad habits, Epstein-Barr, electromagnetic contamination. All of it, sure. But so much already we have edited, gutted, amended.

What is this need for answer. Answer before medication. Am I not a person of faith & action.

I feel it coming. The onset of enough. Of surrender. This is boy's story, too.

x/y

Mimi, boy says at night in bed before I shut his bedroom door before I shut my bedroom door before it is quiet for a few hours before the first scream of night seizure reels.

Mimi, boy says. *Can you give me the medicine.*

What medicine.

The medicine that the doctors say will make my Messis go away.

Give boy Keppra: take boy to epilepsy camp. Could it be: all along White Doctor was right.

x/y

I return to Warhol. To practicality as emotionality. To practicality as practicality. To thoughts of future & prognosis in terms

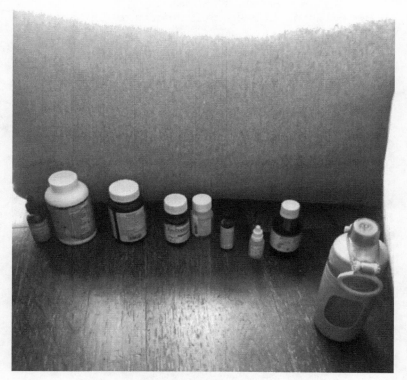

of life lived from viewpoint of six-year-old boy. Thoughts of how long until we give medication. Of why not give. Of what is worse, seizure or medication.

I did as all my witches said. Waited on the medication. Now they say give.

I think to explain to boy the difference between medicine & medication. I think of the difference, this difference, upon which I insist. So much. Upon. What is it really. Medicine vs. medication. Give the body what it needs, no. Quanta amassed into correct combination of substance, substance inserted, onset of fun. Idiopathic uncanny usurping laughter gone.

I return to Warhol. To practicality as lamplight. I do as I've always done when I do not know what to do. I read.

Boy has seizures. Medication stops seizures. Give boy medication. Boy is medicated. Boy is seizure free.

x/y

Seven. Six. Five. Four. Three. Two. One.

It is time. Second opinion time. Wheels set in motion when we were admitted into hospital in early March with mildly laughing, seizing boy are spun.

Airplane wheels spin fast, are tucked, then reemerge so we can land.

x/y

We are led by a nurse to an examination room.

I am going to provoke a seizure we can record, she says. *So doctor can observe it before you meet with him later today. I need to put this blue cap on boy. It's basically an* EEG. *Then I'll use various methods to provoke the seizure. Okay.*

Okay.

First, I'll start with a strobe light.

She turns off the light in the room, then illuminates boy's face with a bright strobe light for some thirty seconds. No seizure comes.

Next she gives boy a pinwheel to blow on. Boy blows. Seizure comes. Bad seizure. Worst Nelson David and I have ever seen.

Three red roses, nurse loudly, repeatedly, says. *Three red roses. Three red roses.*

After some thirty seconds, seizure passes.

Nurse says to boy, *do you remember anything I said.*

No.

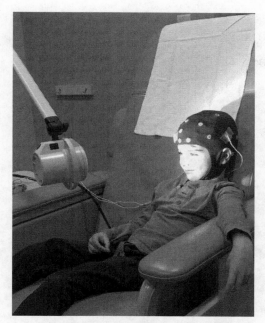

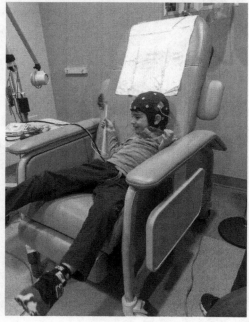

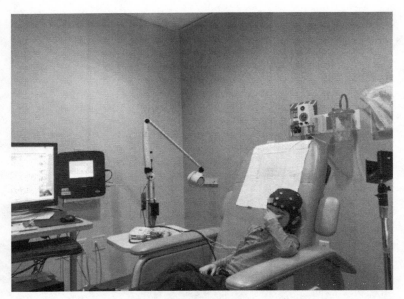

Go grab something to eat if you like. Be at the neurology floor at one to sign in. I got what I needed. That went really well.

x/y

    threeredroses
    three
    red
    roses
    threeredrosesthree
    redrosesthreeredroses threeredroses   three   redroses are
    like a rose is

x/y

How could Simic, so realistic, so metaphysic, so idiomatic, so stanzaic, so ungovernably Slavic, say that having a soul makes no difference.

Feeling literary is the feeling of poem & the feeling of soul. Listening to Leonard Cohen and reading Simic is that, that feeling of soul. Same soul of snuggle puff at night with night-seizing boy.

Soul is not the whole day. The whole day is work. The whole day is company to feed and nothing to say. The whole day is not book. But it is book, day distilled via book into book, that matters, that makes a difference.

Book of experience of seizures of boy makes the difference. Book, soul, access to feeling literary about it all.

If not.   Boy seizes,   is rapt.

What's it to   me.

What's it to

                 you.
                 Rapture un-   written

                               elapsed.

x/y

We wait for our neurologist, Doctor Payne. Payne, Bravo, Columbus, Cruz, Simic, Sergio, Eliot, Elsa, Hamer, Richard, Jonathan, Lispector, Nelly, Lucy, Vet, Cuban Doctor, Warhol, Wonka.

Who else will join our carbon-based cast of stars.

I write down names to review, to revise, our recent past.

Boy, too, decides to write on dry-erase board in medical examination room. A story. He says he is writing a story. We've never seen him try to write a story. What a time to write his first.[29]

O, boy. O, Freud. What sense to make of words.

x/y

I'm not sure why they didn't run an epilepsy protocol on boy's MRI, Dr. Payne says.

What do you mean.

Usually, when you are dealing with a case of potential epilepsy, a neurologist will order an epilepsy protocol on the MRI, *very thin slices of the brain. The slices they took when you were in the hospital are thick. But based on what I am seeing, I am pretty sure boy has dysplasia.*

Dysplasia. After we received the medical reports where dysplasia is listed as a possible cause of the seizures, we met with our neurologist. He said that there was no dysplasia. That actually there was nothing at all in boy's brain. That the MRI *was totally clear.*

No. It's not. Here, see, this cell formation over here. Gives me suffi-cient comfort to call a dysplasia diagnosis and recommend you start boy on medication right away. Did they explain dysplasia to you.

I guess. Sort of.

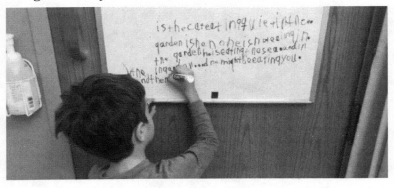

---

29 Is the cat eating quiet in the garden. Is he. No he is not eating in the garden. He is eating the sea. And in the (in) garden he might be eating you. And then he was in the bottom of the sea.

Well, it's basically a moment[30] of disordered growth of the cells of the brain. It happens in utero.[31] For an instant, the cells form in disarray, then they settle back into normal growth patterns. That moment of disarray leaves a scar-type tissue behind that is called dysplasia. Dysplasia usually has a sudden onset at around the age boy has, with sharply escalating seizures. So even clinically, it is a highly plausible diagnosis.

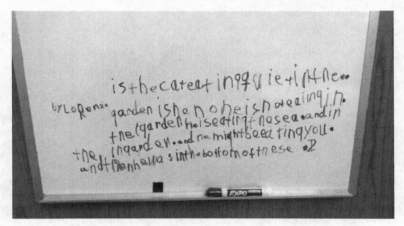

What are the risks. What does this mean for future of boy.

Dysplasia is non-degenerative. It usually doesn't grow or change throughout a person's lifetime. That being said, this type of epilepsy is known as structural epilepsy. This means that it is also very unlikely to go away. There is a less than five percent chance that boy will grow out of his dysplasia-related seizures.

We are struck silent. An answer. An immediate answer. Doctor goes on.

The greatest risk with dysplasia is that it can be resistant to medication. I have three or so medications we can try though, working to adjust the dosages until we get it right. There are also other options we can

---

30 (Event!)

31 In utero. Stab me with those words.

consider at a later date if medication does not work. There are surgeries that remove the dysplasia from the brain. We can also try CBD.

We were given Keppra, but we are working closely with alternative doctors who advise against it due to its toxicity.

We can start boy on something called Trileptal. There are people who've been on it for forty years or so without any negative effects. It's a highly studied drug.

Okay. Why not try CBD off the bat.

It's just so new. We simply don't know yet what CBD will do to a kid's brain, a human brain, after forty years. The Keto diet is also great for treating epilepsy. But, to really have an effect, you need to follow it religiously and monitor boy's blood, draw blood very frequently. I'd advise against this, unless medication doesn't work.

Do you think we need to do another MRI.

Based on what I am seeing, I am pretty confident about this diagnosis. Boy would clearly need general anesthesia to sit still during a forty-minute MRI. Not sure you want to put him under, if you just went through it a few months ago.

No. We don't. We are tired. So is boy. What about genetic testing. Were you able to look at the genetic test we ran. Do we need to run more tests.

Yes, I saw the test. Don't do anymore. The truth is we won't know what to do with the results. The tests I saw merely indicate that boy has mutations on two genes linked to epilepsy. Of course, given the reality, we interpret that to mean that boy has predisposition for epilepsy. But the results don't give us more than that.

We nod. We nod. We nod.[32]

I am going to write a prescription for Trileptal. Go to the pharmacy

---

32 Yes. Yes. Yes.

downstairs & start him on it right away. I'll start you on a very low dose from where we can build. Email me tomorrow and let me know how it goes. We can adjust the dosage before you go home.

Are there any side-effects.

I don't anticipate boy having any. Slight exhaustion is most likely one.

We laugh. Boy is jumping off examination bed. Has not stopped moving since doctor came in room.

What do you think about video games, changes in diet. Could this have any effect on boy's seizures.

There are kids out there who will have seizures from gluten, from dairy. Also, the stimulation from video games can cause seizures, no doubt. A strobe light is one of the ways we tried to provoke a seizure this morning, after all. But, based on all I've seen, again, I feel confident saying his is a case of structural epilepsy. One whose seizures may be activated by external triggers but whose underlying cause is built-in.

Okay. Within this structural epilepsy are there any dietary recommendations. Anything else we should do.

Obviously, he is an active kid. Sugar is not great in general. For anybody. Much less so for a hyperactive kid. So, if you already cut back on that, keep it up. But, honestly, if the medication works, he can go back to a fully normal life.

What if medication doesn't work.

We try others. Others I don't like as much but that are still solid, viable options. Let's just start.

x/y

A name. Not epithet, not blanket, not nickname, not perhaps.

Not idio/pathic.

But fact.

But now.

We hasten to obtain substance to insert.

All we will, all we say, is medication, please, just, work.

x/y

It happens on or around Week Six. The embryo by then is formed of three layers: ectoderm, mesoderm, endoderm: outer, middle, inner. From Week Six on, we are beings of layers. It is the ectoderm that develops into brain & skin. Mesoderm turns into bones, ligaments, reproductive organs. Endoderm cells become intestines, lungs.

Ectoderm cells progress, by time of birth, into the mediators of body's interactions with external world: skin and brain. Touch & apprehend.

When construction screws up, the errors, as birthmarks— of brain, of skin—show up. Dysplasia. Baffling manifestation of absolute fact, absolute act. It just happens, we say, because we cannot conceive a cause. Effect, though, is clear.

x/y

I write Elsa, *Dysplasia, they say. Trileptal, they say.*

Great, she says. *Trileptal is a great option. Not so toxic. Get on it.*

We get on it. Insert new substance into small boy. Eat dinner, shower, get to bed. Wonder when, if, how, night seizures will emerge.

x/y

This is the chemical composition of Oxcarbazepine, the generic name of Trileptal: $C_{15}H_{12}N_2O_2$. Here is what its molecule looks like:

Levetiracetam, also known as Keppra, is this: $C_8H_{14}N_2O_2$.

One more hydrogen, five more carbon. But, fundamentally, essentially, the same atoms. Same vacuum between subatomic parts. Different arrangement. Different amalgam. Out of soup comes flop, sop. But. Out of this same celestial soup comes opus. Dose & antidote conveyed to us by anagram.[33]

x/y

We wake. Wake & are rested.

Did you hear anything, we say. *No. Nothing. Something minor round six am. Something like a dubious sneeze. But really. Nothing.*

We monitor throughout the day. Take boy to place where he can run and play. Write doctor, tell him no seizures so far today.

Write Elsa, tell her from fifteen to twenty, no seizures so far today. She says, *Amen to the work of the hand of God.*

x/y

Intentionally, incidentally, left blank—

———

33 Whitman in line three of "Song of Myself" says:

For every atom belonging to me as good belongs to you.

How much more do we know now than what Whitman back then guessed.

9

Perhaps to gather, encircle, Nina Real back within this story-
ring of usurped boy, I embark on search for Eliot's children's
book of verse: '*Old Possum's Book of Practical Cats.*' A book to
share with her, only her, her: only daughter, whose only parents absent from her realm of real because of parallel, non-over-
lapping, sequence of seizing sibling boy.[34]

At the bookstore, I do not find '*Old Possum's Book*' on its
own. Instead, I am handed part two of a two-part anthology of
Eliot's complete poems less capacious volume, lies '*Practical Cats
and Further Verse.*'

I start with "Macavity: The Mystery Cat". Circle on to
"The Rum Tug Tugger", hoping to round out with "The
Naming of Cats." But, by then, I've lost her. Nina Real is not
drawn in, drawn toward Eliot's heroic, tragic, ecstatic, the-
atric *killy* cats. She is distracted, wants to play, her the mommy,
me the baby *killy* cat.

I am never too tired to read. But, often, am too tired, utterly
drained, to play. To pretend. Can I just be me myself, mother
in her bed, reading her a book instead.[35] Perhaps. But not this
book. I reach for others: Clifford, Peppa, her darling Grinch.

She is drawn, trapped, and I am grateful. It is the drawings.
Their lines, their colors: lures that allure. Patterns, like magic,
that perform the charge of pretend.

---

34 *Am I not here with you, I who am your mother.*
35 *Am I not here with you, I who am your mother.*

( )

We are sent home from second opinion hospital with white substance (bottled and inserted) & non-seizing six-year-old boy. Less than twenty-four hours after we start lowest dose of medication, seizures cease.

Nothing more. *Nada más.*

What we have is both neatness & extravagance conveyed via document: "dysplasia" stamped upon a medical clinical report. That classic, elusive moment of truth, recorded. "Medication," "diagnosis," "prognosis," "attenuation": words I presume, now, to use.

I enjoy boy's medical clinical report passionately, quote by quote. Embrace it in my temporary hands. A golden ticket. My relief full, full as

	echo	that I hurl
from here—	toward the round	drum
	of your soul.	

( )

(soul…soul…soul…)

( )

Annaya is name of physical place in Lebanon. Place where Lebanon's Catholic patron saint, Saint Charbel, had his hermitage: today a place of pilgrimage.

Saint Charbel is a busy saint.[36] One invoked often on behalf of Anaya, my friend's now twenty-five-month daughter diagnosed with stage four cancer. In reading about Saint Charbel, I discover that Anglican spelling of place is not Anaya, like daughter. But rather Annaya, or Annaaya, or Aannaya.

In Spanish *ya* is both "already" and "now." Ana/ya a way to say "Ana/already/now."

Ana ya. Ana now.
Already.

A connection to my name, my native tongue, that I casually considered, that I unconcernedly liked. A connection that I am concerned to discover is not.

It's just not.

What I do find: *Anaya*, the meaning behind word that serves as name, when internet delved, throws—

Answer of God.

( )

An answer. Give the mind what it wants, no. An answer. A term both noun & verb, like circle, like hand, like throw.

Below is Merriam-Webster's answer to question of how word lands as noun—

---

36 *The Economist* published article in 2018 chronicling increase of miracles attributed to St. Charbel in Lebanon. Miracles on the rise it says. Is miracle a thing akin to self-fulfilling prophecy. What has happened once, more than once, can surely happen again, for us. Surely it will. So surely it does.

an·swer | \ 'an(t)-sər \

1. a: something spoken or written in reply to a question
   His answer surprised us.
   b: a correct response knows the *answer*
2. a reply to a legal charge or suit: PLEA
   also: DEFENSE
3. something done in response or reaction
   His only answer was to walk out.
4. a solution of a problem
   More money is not the answer.
5. one that imitates, matches, or corresponds to another
   The show is television's answer to the news magazines.

( )

Prions were discovered, first named, by Dr. Stanley Prusiner, the 1997 Nobel Prize-winning, still-living Director of the Institute for Neurodegenerative Diseases at the University of California in San Francisco.[37] On the site of Nobel Prize, Dr. Prusiner describes his life, the findings that resulted in prize, the persistent doubts, despite—

"While it is quite reasonable for scientists to be skeptical of new ideas that do not fit within the accepted realm of scientific knowledge, the best science often emerges from situations where results carefully obtained do not fit within the accepted paradigms. At times the press became involved since the media provided the naysayers with a means to vent their frustration at not being able to find the cherished nucleic acid that they were so sure must exist."

---

37 Prions, self-replicating protein particles that can cause cells of brain to become sponge-like. Prions that are generally found in all of our bodies but can go rogue, for reasons unknown: prions cause mad cow disease.

The *"accepted paradigm"* to which Dr. Prusiner refers is this—

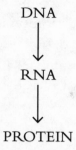

DNA

RNA

PROTEIN

The name for this chain is *The Central Dogma of Life*. A name given to assembly line of life by Francis Crick, one of three winners of 1962 Nobel Prize in Physiology or Medicine. Prize won for the discovery of molecular structure of DNA: its double-helix ladder, skeleton blueprint, custom craft scaffold to individualized life.[38]

Here is what the University of Utah says about prions & skepticism—

"Ever since Stanley Prusiner coined the term "prion" in 1982 and showed that purified prions can transmit spongiform disease, skeptics have been trying to prove him wrong. The idea that a protein can reproduce itself without going through a nucleic acid intermediate goes against everything we know about transmissible diseases. Even the simplest viruses contain genetic material, DNA or RNA, that codes for proteins necessary for function and transmission. Because prions appear to be infectious proteins that can self-replicate, the central dogma of molecular biology, (DNA to RNA to protein) seems not to apply here."

———

38 First come, first name.

If DNA is keyboard of source, then what is prion. If DNA customizes body's proteins, how do prions go rogue, why.

Why—if by scientific definition, by laboratory observation, by repeated clinical trial, by specialized research—prion is protein, segment of customized life. Protein, but without DNA, without RNA, without nucleic acid, without encoded language of origin, of parent, of propagation. Yet able to propagate, despite.

By definition, then: uncertain if living, if dead. In my own words: undead: zombie splinter of organic matter.

What is cancer. What—if not groups of proteins, cellularly conformed, gone rogue. What is prion. What is cancer. What is rogue.

The internet agrees that a virus cannot self-reproduce. That it needs a host. (Unhappy host!) Internet agrees a virus has an encapsulated strand of nucleic acid, of DNA and/or RNA, that uses nucleus of host to replicate. Viral entity that, by generating more of itself via nucleus of host, causes life curve of host to stray from its track.

Okay.

But as regards self-replication of prions, the internet does not agree. The internet agrees to disagree. Prion is problematic—protein-child of DNA, of RNA, with no memory, no remnant, no imbed of cradle. Source-less material of life. That when rogue exists to kill.

If DNA conveys Lesson, Inescapable Truth of Who We Are. If it paves Way. Then, is virus Axle. Is prion Axis. Is cancer Arc meant to redirect, to resurface, Way.

Is disease pure evil or pure survival, pure intention. Is it measure of will. Will beyond all will. Edifying, unequivocal shove of God.

( )

Violet turned violet turned violet turned violet.

( )

One week after I return home with seizureless boy, I fly to Bogotá, alone. Fly to sign sale of company. Documents prepared while at second opinion hospital. The task of multi-task.

It is swift. Two physical hands sign two material papers & an entity called "company" transfers conceptual ownership hands. It is instant. It is event. It is past.

As it happens, I wonder: is this the place my story of usurped boy will end.

An only happy story. Respite.

( )

Two nights before Anaya dies, I eat with her mother, my friend, while I am coincidentally, incidentally, in New York, where Anaya is preparing for last part of her cancer treatment. Treatment is going so well. Anaya is doing so well. Now it is a waiting game. For her counts to rise. For immunotherapy time.

Being here for treatment has actually been so special, friend says. *I grew up here. The City is home. My mom is here. My sister is here. I'd always wanted to come back for a good chunk of time with my kids. But never had the chance.*

Maybe Anaya brought you here, I say.

Yes. She did. I really do think so. Her illness has fulfilled so many wishes.

What do you mean.

Well, my wish to reconnect with the City. Other wishes I had.

Like what.

My wish to write, for one. I've been writing so much. Just for myself.
It's been my form of therapy. But also, other people's wishes. My moth-
er's wish to have us closer. And, here we are in New York. I've recon-
nected with my sisters. I've even reconnected with music.

It's amazing you can see things this way.

We are so hopeful. Anaya is doing so well. None of the nurses can
believe how brave she is. She offers her arm with a smile before they even
go to draw blood. It's like she just knows.

She is such a warrior. She is going to be fine. I am certain of it. In my
mind, it is a fact.

( )

The first poem, the first   wish,   I ever
                              publish
                              is
                              this—

A Girlfriend for Prufrock

A not small, not ugly, not quiet, unclumsy gal,
Prone to corners, hiccups, sauces and wine.
Occasionally invited,
But, as a guest, addressed only once and not by all.
A woman-child without absolute truths,
Inclined to sit straight, stand slumped and steal stares.
Intuitively clever
But, in delivery, too eager with wit, too late with flair.

The not-lady, not-graceful, not-charming you,
With a lonely métier she says is best left for two:
To self-involve the self-eschewed
In the hollow of a silver spoon.

( )

CHAPTER 9   253

Husband and I converse. All is ready for our trip to go see Cuban Doctor in the florid heat of Guayaquil. Never had we thought boy would be so well. One, two, three, four weeks after second option trip & nothing: not a single electric, somatic, volcanic, magmatic swell, not even a hiccup, not even a flinch.

Do we cancel Guayaquil.

( )

The late afternoon, the early evening, the few hours before dusk on day before day Anaya dies, I go with her mom, my friend, to Leonard Cohen exhibit at New York's Jewish Museum. Here we find a bird on a wire. Filmed, captured, fixed, fixated, upon wall.

Also, a room where you can lie down on benches and put on headphones and hear voices hum Cohen's *Hallelujah* to ya. Afterwards we go get pie at Austrian bakery. I ask cold Austrian waitress for cold Austrian drink and she suggests a cold Almdudler. Of course, we are charmed.

An Almdudler then vs. an Almdudler now. How much do I remember of red boy red girl outlined in white on can. What can I tell you of the ways memory has turned. They are so many, the ways. The turns. I dread when next a red Almdudler intersects the edge of my breadth.

( )

Not the thing, but the combination of, I believe, stopped onslaught of seize. The thing, of course—the medication—science inserted into open mouth of boy. But the preparation, too, of body to receive. The detoxification: of Epstein-Barr, of parasites, of sugar, of gluten, of dairy, of entities, of toxic electromagnetic flood.

I've opened my mouth.[39] Boy opens his mouth.[40] From somewhere—

> The sense our auras, our souls, are not same, are changed.
> I am exhausted. Bled dry. Is it my aura.
> Did it drain out.

( )

Incidentally, the soundtrack of recently medicated, non-seizing boy is this: Portishead's *Dummy*. I begin listening to it convulsively. Seismically. Album introduced to me by Sam, who drove me to high school before I could drive: she a senior, I a low freshman girl.

Sam played *Dummy* over and over again in the mornings of my freshman year, mornings spent in her white Toyota Corolla, a personable land that smelled of tree-shaped, rear-view-mirror air freshener, open cans of Diet Coke and Parliament cigarette smoke.

Out of nowhere—the desire for this music comes. I hunt for it. Load it down onto my electric, magnetic device. It is music that serves generous literary purposes. Music that I alternate with Sting's *Sad Trombone*.

Music that is good to write to, good to work to, good to have good coffee to. Music that becomes the same as onset of non-convulsive day-to-day real world. This world in which I walk and am a mother whose boy does not quiver, does not quake, does not shiver—oh no, good God—he does not shake.

( )

---

39 To say.
40 To take.

On the day Anaya dies these lines are cut as text:

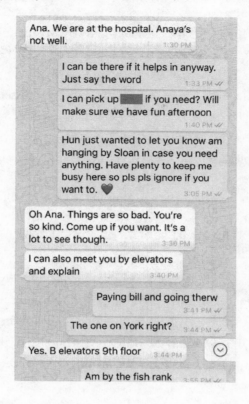

> **Ana. We are at the hospital. Anaya's not well.** 1:30 PM
>
> I can be there if it helps in anyway. Just say the word 1:33 PM ✓✓
>
> I can pick up ▮▮▮ if you need? Will make sure we have fun afternoon 1:40 PM ✓✓
>
> Hun just wanted to let you know am hanging by Sloan in case you need anything. Have plenty to keep me busy here so pls pls ignore if you want to. 🖤 3:05 PM ✓✓
>
> **Oh Ana. Things are so bad. You're so kind. Come up if you want. It's a lot to see though.** 3:36 PM
>
> **I can also meet you by elevators and explain** 3:40 PM
>
> Paying bill and going therw 3:41 PM ✓✓
>
> The one on York right? 3:44 PM ✓✓
>
> **Yes. B elevators 9th floor** 3:44 PM
>
> Am by the fish rank 3:55 PM ✓✓

( )

It's happening.

( )

When I finished reading *For Whom the Bell Tolls,* I hurled the book from my bed. I wanted to launch the story away, get it physically off of me. Expunge it. Delete it. For days, I was violently pissed at Hemingway. Fucking big-game-hunting, alcoholic Hemingway. Why not keep your misery to yourself,

Ernest. *Pero por Diós, Ernesto, por qué.* Why write this skull of a
story. Why sit so still to will it out.

A story that is not fact. A fiction. Why invent such sad fiction when sad is such fact.

Yet. I knew the story, the book, was based on the witnessed
wars of his life, actual wars, actual life. I was not pissed at fiction
but wrecked by fact.

All stories are fiction are fact. Everything always possible,
always tellable, simultaneously, at once. What is the difference.
Between fuck, between fax, between fact. How many letters
separate each word. How many rungs. Is what we hold not the
same as what we throw.

That the bell tolls it tolls.

( )

What theory do you use for cancer patient baby in hospital
with sudden active hemorrhage in brain. In terms of semiotics
is blood the signifier, hemorrhage the signified. Together with
what are they sign, is it together with slit, with slice, with split
thin cranial vein.

What ultimate understanding of ultimate reality of life
applies. What hokey pokey. What vacuum. What prayer. Blood
in brain if it flows out too fast has nowhere to go. This I know
from father. My father with blood in the brain going into operating room for doctors to drain. Brain can only soak up so much
blood loose from its veins.

Am I here to document the passionate moment, the instant,
the event, when friend's baby has precipitous stroke. The rapture. The appearing & disappearing. The aftermath of interim.
The mathematics of after. Will it exact subtraction.

Am I here to record how it feels to have friend before me, sitting before me, friend whose baby has still-flowing stroke. Friend who knows. Am I here to bear witness. I think of Nelly, who on her Reiki table had said, the purpose, lesson, of seizures, of all this, is poem.

A coincidence I am here. An incident. An experience into which I am thrown.

Here, to document the massive loss of single two-year-old child. The shock of sudden, always sudden, no matter how rigorous the disease.

Here, to sit next to young mother who knows. Young mother who says, *baby's father keeps positive, but I can no longer ignore the facts*. By the fish tank of the ninth-floor children's cancer research ward, young mother before me, sitting in front, cannot, can no longer look me in eye. The look will confirm what she knows. What I, too, know. We know. We look away, at the tank, its fish: fisheyes look at us straight because what they cannot know they cannot fear to say.

( )

Oh, Anne, Professor Anne, Professor Carson, Anaya is dying. You, who knows all the myths, all the acts of appearing & disappearing, you—

Please: tell me, what can I write to make it stop.

( )

Oh Ana.

( )

If I were to write the character of Jo/ana, not the thing but the combination of, Jonathan & Ana, not of Lispector's Joana, but of our Joana, what would she read like.

Not like Lispector's.

Lispector's Joana for whom all stories begin continuously, incessantly, at once: in the now: now—from whence all may be written, all may be erased, equally, at once.

But Jonathan & Ana is a timorous coy girl. Our Jo/ana moves forward but submits, bows, tenders to edit. Edit of strikethrough, mess of indelible pen.

Her words, incidentally, sound similar to words I've said in this book. To what I believe I believe. About brain about mind about good coffee. About God & Bible & Quixote & sad. About how sad is a manuscript cupped by two hands.

What I think I want to believe.

Lispector's Joana is able to disregard what life reveals because she doesn't care about lesson. Only living matters, a living so fascinating there is no room for despair. Her experience always hovers above, a play that outplays any sad facts of time & space.

But Jonathan & Ana. We care. We care about what the past becomes, of what becomes of the past. Of the story. Because we are bound, we stay. We survey, we consider, and, with effort, we take pain to say.

( )

We cannot depend on others to stay alive, I say to friend who calls for update on baby from hospital waiting room.

I am unable to know I think this before I say this.

We have to cultivate our own garden, I say. Old quote from old Voltaire's old *Candide*. Who am I that says such a blank, such a

feeble, such a pathetic thing. Do I not control even the things
I say.

This feels like death, I say. *Seeing mother of baby's face feels like
death,* I say.

Do not go there, friend on phone says. *We cannot go there. Baby
is at hospital used to dealing with this sort of thing.*

My father had blood in the brain, I say. *They drained it. They
cannot drain baby's brain. Her platelets are too low. They cannot open
her. They are giving her healthy blood through existing, previously open
IV. Hoping new blood will improve her blood so body can close the vein.*

Out loud, I do not go there, go into who emerged from
paternal drain of brain. Not father, not *papi.* Who as whom.
We hang up. But I am already there. A where that is nowhere
but there.

I go downstairs. Find the hospital coffee shop. Again, it is
at once a Starbucks but also, immediately, not. I cannot drink
from this cup, this cup of hospital linked to past, to hopeful
baby cups.

I go outside. Hunt for coffee on medical clinical upper York
Ave. Find a place that is not Starbucks. Drink unlike cup.

( )

Come back to me, Beloved, or I die!

( )

Dr. Camilo Cruz, of thirty-six self-help book fame, fulfills the
airplane-neighbor promise made. Cruz emails me picture of
letter written by Mexican writer Juan Rulfo to his wife, from
book which Cruz discovers in a bookstore in the colonial square
of Usaquén in Bogotá. Book we'd discussed on plane ride back

from my Spring Break Witch Doctor Bogotá 2019 Tour. What
Dr. Cruz says, he does.

In turn, I had mentioned a book I had discovered at another
Bogotá bookstore, La Tornamesa, which houses a stirring selection of books in Spanish for children. My book a kid's book by
Lispector about a chicken named Laura, called *The Intimate Life
of Laura.*

Rulfo's letter is a present to plunder. In it Rulfo tells his wife
her mouth tastes like stolen sugar, and her cheeks like the heart's
memory of peach. Not the thing, but memory of.

Rulfo closes his letter with this—

"I am hurry because finished me the ink."

His letter written in Spanish save for this last line, this dead-
line. Does English serve finality better. Stipulation, discipline,
bespeak. Finished me. The ink.

I too am hurry. Finishing me, the ink. These memories of
life, when put on paper, I feel them: they are relieved. Despite
hurt, there is relief. Relief of memory that almost slipped.

( )

We decide to go to Guayaquil. Why. Why do we decide to go
to Guayaquil.

( )

Craving is to hunger as

          epigenetics is to genetics.
It is not a versus relationship. But one
    of   beyond.
One of evolve. One of   hop on top. One
of combination
        of.

One of wish,
of fancy, of yearn, of become. Be   come
versus   be,

                    aspire versus need.

( )

Sam, amiga Sam: sad I am.

Baby Anaya died, Sam. She did not make it to freshman year, to morning light and luminous numinous Parliament cigarette smoke.

"In loving memory of Anaya." Reads the plaque on park bench a group of friends join to inscribe. I am asked to write the plaque. I sit down to write it in front of gate for flight home from New York. I compose options for group of friends to decide—

1.
Sit here & sit with me;
Go & also go with me.
'In loving memory
of Anaya.'

2.
Sit here & sit with me;
Go & also go with me.
In memory of Anaya,
One of love & jubilee.

3.
Sit here & sit with me;
Go & also go with me.
Here we celebrate Anaya
In loving, joyful memory

I stand up to board flight. I miss flight. Flight is closed. Has closed. All are aboard. But I can no longer board. It is too late. All aboard. Airline attendant looks at me. Has seen me stand up from gate seat and walk ten feet to board. To not board. Does not ask. Does not say.

Is there another flight.

Yes. I will get you on. It's in an hour. Go straight to the gate. Please, just be sure to board.

( )

Less than five percent of all cases of dysplasia see seizures disappear. Numerically, our chances look like this: <5%.

Trileptal has been around for decades. People have taken it for decades. Boy can take it for decades. No problem. Seizures are gone. Every morning and night we draw two ml's into syringe & insert substance into boy's mouth.

Problem solved.

( )

What happens to Mary after Jesus dies. Of Mary I know— her suffering. Her suffering at feet of dying son. Then, centuries later, her apparitions. Out of thin air—Mary—phantom, specter, like a narrow arrow blade. The millions drawn toward, drawn by. Circumscribed by her plight.

Churches, chapels, basilicas, cathedrals built. For her. For her suffering. Her evanescence. Monuments of aspirational salvation built for grace of maternal love. Notre-Dame. Our Lady of Guadalupe. Our Lady of Chiquinquira. Steeples risen, vaulted gothic domes arisen, glass rosettes to adorn the story of a mother and her single boy.

What is Mary if not that infinitely suffering, infinitely gentle, thing of which Eliot in his 'Preludes' spoke. Do we flock to this notion, this fancy, when we flock to Mary. Gentle internal suffering, idealized. Materialized. Externalized. Popularized. Generalized. And so, finally, neutralized.

There, Mary, upon that altar: if she is that eternally suffering, eternally gentle thing, then that thing, for a moment, for an instant, can no longer be me.

( )

Boy is fine. Can I say. Dare I. Boy is well. Even with medication, his change is to us as Elsa says, the work of the hand of God. We remain at lowest possible dose of medication. Weeks pass, ceaselessly seizure-free. Do I say it. I do. Precipitously seizure-free is miraculous but also eerie, uncanny: unheimlich as fax.

( )

We tell boy about Anaya. He is confused. He doesn't understand. We try to explain. Her brain was tired. So many treatments. The disease was strong. I employ parataxis. Short declarative sentences. For intended effect. Effect of juvenile explain.

But boy does not get. It.

What don't you get, I finally say, surprised, immediately ashamed, at my impatience, or is it my rage. *She was sick. She passed away.*

Mimi. But she was in the hospital. How can you die if you are in a hospital.

( )

I speak to friend, mom of Lionel. I say: *tell me what to say. Please. Is there anything you wish you would have heard when it happened, anything anyone could've said right away.*

No, there is nothing. It's all shock. The one thing I frantically wanted to read was the poem by Chanel Brenner, 'A Poem for Women Who Don't Want Children,' the one you shared with me years ago.

Yes. I did. I sent it.

Okay.

What about after. In the weeks to come. What should I do. After.

Well a new baby is important. But don't tell her that. It's obvious and so hard.

Is there anything I can ever do, ever say.

Someone asked me if the experience of losing Lionel changed me. It took me a while to figure it out. But, basically, I had to relearn everything. Everything was new. My house was new. Walking was new. Because this was now a world where your baby can die. So I wasn't different but the world was different.

Is there anything that brought you comfort.

It was really hard explaining things to Lionel's brother. There's a book that helped. It even helped me. Maybe you can get that for Anaya's brother. It's about lifespans of different animals. Just how lifespans are all different. Live the lifespan of a turtle vs. the lifespan of a dragonfly. Some of us just have a different lifespan.

Okay. Anything else.

The suddenness of how Lionel died eventually became sort of comforting. I know Anaya was sick, but her death still seems so sudden. As a parent, suddenness is horribly shocking, but if it means your kid doesn't suffer, you take that deal.

How did you make it through.

Well, you have to. So you do.

( )

Two weeks after Anaya dies, we take off. Wheels spin, are spun. Round and round and round: over and over & over again. Airplane flies south to Guayaquil.

Why we tell ourselves, other selves, we go—

- Perhaps Cuban Doctor's treatments can find a more holistic way of eliminating seizures. A way not dependent upon medication.
- Boy is challenging to parent. Hyper/over/active. Could dysplasia evolve into ADHD as pediatrician months before said. Surely, we can help calm boy's impulsivity with whatever there is in Guayaquil.
- Improve upon <5% of course perhaps why not.
- We will have to evaluate dosages each year. Be wary of break-through seizures. This means a medical clinical life. Could Guayaquil eradicate seizures for good.

Why we go—

- F/H
- E/O
- A/P
- R/E

( )

Guayaquil is a colorless place. Decolored. Discolored. Illegible place. With a brown winding river shore beneath ashen overcast humid sky. I'm so sorry if you are from Guayaquil but it is a place that is brown and gray and clammy everywhere like broken mud brick. It is nowhere a belly button always a gut. We go to hospital. Many children in waiting room. Boy is miserable. He feels he's been tricked. This he feels because

he has. We made up some evil lie about going to soccer camp
in Guayaquil. Being parent turns you into liar. The price to
be paid for this. To make things easier, I've read up on history
of world wars. To tell to boy during treatment. Two hours
each day for twenty days. To captivate boy. A doctor sees boy.
Cuban Doctor's son. We ask why set up shop here in this mono-
chrome place. Cuban Doctor's son talks only of Cuba. Of joy
of Cuba. Of leaving Cuba and not having joy because Cuba is
talk and music and dance and joy. Nowhere else is this. All this
talk while he preps boy. Boy is not breathing well is hyper-
ventilating so they play a movie on TV in prep room and boy
calms down although boy doesn't watch TV really only soccer
and ninja obstacle courses and science videos. And TV is dubbed
in bad dubbed Spanish and I am writing all that is happening
into the back of whatever book I am reading at time and I can't
remember now what book it was. I've looked for the book
through my recent books through stacks of books to find what
I wrote but no sign of book not in my stacks nor in my memory
of this time. And then son of Cuban Doctor is done and Cuban
Doctor comes in and they turn off TV while Cuban Doctor runs
scan and is done with scan and says I cannot treat boy. I am sorry
so sorry you came all this way but I cannot treat boy. Not here
not now not anywhere. Why of course we say. Why. But why.
We came all this way. Because his brain is convulsed. His electromagnetic waves are off are identical to those of seizing brain.
But we say he's been so well we almost canceled our trip he's
been so well. It's unbelievable how well he's been. Could it be
anti-seizure medication. Also he's had a cough and we've given
cough syrup could it be that. No. None of that. None of what
you could give could change brain waves like that. Perhaps
boy is nervous. Look at how he breathes. If I start treatment

he might seize. I cannot risk that. I will give you your money
back and you can go home. Is there anything else we can do. His
iron is still too low. You need to increase it. I would do a heavy
metals test. But already we are giving him iron supplements
though we understand it takes time for blood to absorb. Also
we did the metal heavy test. Here are the results. Look. Here.
We went over them already with doctors with Elsa. They said
there is not much in boy's blood. There is some silver, Cuban
Doctor says. His silver is almost at seventy percent. Silver in the
blood together with low iron could make it harder for him to
obtain oxygen. Make him breath like that. Also anxiety. Look I
turn on the TV and he is calm. Treat his nerves. Clean his blood.

( )

In Burton's *Charlie and the Chocolate Factory*, repeatedly, compulsively, watched by Nina Real, there is scene in which Willy
Wonka takes Charlie Bucket and Mike Teavee to room where
Wonka and the Oompa Loompas have discovered how to
deliver chocolate by television screen. A magic lantern, if you
will, that throws chocolate morsels onto patterns on a screen.

   Mike Teavee screams at Wonka. Claims Wonka has just
invented the first teleportation machine in the history of
humankind. Claims Wonka does not understand what Wonka
has invented. Claims Wonka does not understand the difference
between particles & waves. Despite the Wonka chocolate bar
teleportation haze above his and Charlie Bucket's heads.[41]

------

41   It is only in Burton's version that Mike Teavee shouts and says *Wonka
     does not understand the difference between particles and waves.* Line is not
     in book. Not in Gene Wilder movie. Is there a seepage of particle,
     of wave into popular culture, into collective mind that is recently
     imperative. I gather. Because of seepage of question we now see it on
     page, page of Burton's movie script. Because seepage, page.

I cannot get scene outside my head. Do I understand the difference between particles & waves. Do I.

It seems like difference I, traversing this specific, narrative, sequence of life events, should understand. I look online. Go to physics forums. Define the difference, the question, in my own words. In words I own.

A particle, I gather, is this: the last bit of chocolate that is still chocolate. But, particle is also this: endless universe of small. The splicing of chocolate molecule into parts. And so on forever: forever everything theoretically labeled into parts. Forever not the thing: eternally the combination of. From what I gather, I gather this: eventually when a thing, a particle, gets so small it behaves no different than wave, than tremor of energy condensed as memory of place.

Wave is trickier yet to enclose. Perhaps a wave is this: a pull or push but not the thing that flows. Movement of energy without movement of matter. A measurement of surge. Not the water of the river but its motion, its gush, its course. Wind, gravity, full moon but not the water that rises, not the substance, just its force.

Yet: the river, its current. How are they not the same. From where I stand, I see not particle vs. river but water as wave.

Electromagnetic I believe means this: particle and its impulse; present, pressing proclivity of matter described by amplitude of wave.

Boy's electromagnetic fields are off. His flow. His particles, his waves, channels of transfer amiss within his physical head.

( )

Silver in boy's blood. Silver from the nebulae.

( )

Boy is ashamed embarrassed by his epilepsy. He refuses to read book on epilepsy given by beloved sister-in-law. Refuses, that is, to read it in front, even, of beloved cousin Sebastian, of Nina Real. Breathes off, hyperventilates, when asked about disease, about MRI, about CT Scan. But wants to read epilepsy book every night, compulsively, alone with me.

Mimi, he says when we are in Guayaquil. *You forgot my book. My epilepsy book.*

So far sole focus has been physical: emotional stress of disease unexplored. Boy is so well. Except for this, his breathing sometimes feels foreign, feels off. Do I let it slide[42] or do I pursue new rabbit hole. Oh God, could it be: effed up heart behavior.

( )

Am I writing a story that is not mine to write. Am I no better: first come, first name. Does story belong to boy. To Lionel. To Anaya. Should I ask if anyone minds. I do. I ask. No. That's a lie. I don't ask. I tell. *I am writing this story,* I say. *You're in it,* I say. *I'll send it to you.*

If story is not mine. Whose. What's your story about. When asked, I am not sure I know. Not story of sad. Jesus. Not that. At least. Not just that. God. I need a coffee. Quote by quote. There is something I approach. Something else I miss. I circle back. My head a heavy ball.

Being happy is for what.

( )

---

42 See Chapter 5.

Day before we leave Guayaquil, I go to Cuban Doctor's office to pick up printed report. To pick up our full refund.

When I go to leave woman at front desk says, *wait, another mother with daughter is headed your way. Share a taxi.*

Okay.

We climb into taxi. Mother, daughter, myself.

Hi, I am Ana.

Hi. Maria José. This is my daughter.

Are you Colombian.

Yes, we are from Bogotá.

I try to say hi to girl to daughter but realize she cannot, will not, say.

How old is she.

She is six.

My boy is six, too. Have you been coming here long.

A few years. At first, we came for two months at a time, every two or three months. But it was too much. I'd come here alone with her and though she got better I went home each time a wreck. Now we come three times per year.

This place is so weird. There is something about it. It's just off.

Yes. It totally is. But the treatment has helped us so much.

Really. Tell me please.

My daughter could not walk, could not stand when we started coming here. Could not say a word. Now she walks and, though only I & her father can understand her, she communicates, almost talks.

That's wonderful. We are getting sent back. Doctor says my boy's brain is in convulsive state. Boy has epilepsy, but it's still so strange. He's been so well. Hasn't seized in months, not since we started medication in May. We are so confused and a bit in shock.

I am so sorry. I am sure you were so hopeful, one has to be so hopeful, to come here. Doctor is very responsible. He must have his reasons. I've seen the kids he treats recover in miraculous ways. I know most of the moms who come. One mom I know well, her daughter used to seize over one hundred times per day. No medications worked. She had to come for treatment several times but in the end, her daughter's seizures fully stopped. Her daughter must be ten now and leads a normal life. Maybe you can come back.

I don't know. But, yes, perhaps. Can I ask you what your daughter has.

I don't know. No one does. We've tried everything. Still. She remains undiagnosed.

We are quiet. Maria José peels a clementine for her daughter to have. The smell is too bright for the brown grey car.

Take my number, she says. Call me if you decide to come back. I know all the good places to go with kids. Make the experience as good as can be.

Thank you. That would be great. I have to say you are amazing for coming here so much.

The things one does for love.[43]

( )

Guaya   quil.
Place
we go   to leave.

( )

To spool my mind/soul/aura back in from brown grey fog of Guayaquil, sudden tragic passing of baby Anaya, months of seismic boy, strain of lawsuit, of sale of company—what to do

---

43   *(Las cosas que uno hace por amor.)*

but consume fresh words that will spill/seep into me. What to do but read.

I select Dr. Oliver Sacks, *Gratitude*. Not at all the breed of book I tend to read but am drawn toward, encircled by it because: it is swansong. Last essays, final only happy stories written by a revolutionarily kind man before he passed. But also: it is short. Forty-five pages. A double shot espresso of what should be solid longing.[44] I am beset by impatient funk.

In the book, I read this:

> Francis Crick[45] was convinced that "the hard problem"—understanding how the brain gives rise to consciousness—would be solved by 2030.

I become happy when I read this. At least, I laugh. 2030. The hard problem. Ha. Understand the root of all consciousness, its how. Ha. To say we hope to understand consciousness is same as to say we hope to understand cloud—observational facts of behavior/formation are not knowledge of origination. In other words, do you lay your hand upon fire based upon your faith in the weather report.

Quote by quote no revelatory beads are strung. Yet around my neck recent events are hung. I shoulder their weight. They matter. But I cannot say they are matter. Did anything happen. Into boy's mouth cloud-white medication goes. Not even sure of what this matter does.

( )

---

44 Few words are adjectives, adverbs, nouns & verbs. "Long" is one. To long so long for longing that is long.

45 Crick, as in Nobel prizer, first comer, first namer, of the *Central Dogma of Life*.

The following is non-dialectic transcript of boy's air-thrown words in car on way to consult with child psychologist who will tell if boy has trauma, PTSD, related to epilepsy—

Tell me about baby Anaya.

I know it's not an only happy story.

Where does cancer come from.

How can a baby get cancer.

What types of cancer are there.

What did they do to baby Anaya to make her get better.

Why didn't it work.

How did the cancer kill her.

Why couldn't they fix the bleeding.

Why couldn't they give her new blood.

What's radiation.

What's chemotherapy.

Tell me about the Titanic.

In a science video.

I know that's also not happy.

Why did it sink.

What's an iceberg.

Why didn't they see it.

Why don't they float.

Why were people not rescued.

Why didn't we just go to second hospital.

Why didn't we just go to second hospital where they made my Messis go away.

Stopping the sugar did not stop the Messis.

What does sugar do that is bad.

You gave me sugar so Messis are your fault.

( )

For Nina Real, that sleepyhead, I find lovesong.[46] A mariachi morning song: not mine, but ours. You see, she has two moles above her upper lip. Tiny dots, by an unknown hand, perfectly drawn. Two dots that are planetary in size, loci of nuclear self-combustion, suns.

You see, there is a mariachi song that from growing up with mariachi-loving father (this particular, remarkable assemblage of particles) is song that I, too, learned to love. It is called 'Cielito Lindo': little lovely sky. However, *cielo*, or "sky," is term of endearment in Spanish. *Mi cielo*, "my sky," my dear. So, figuratively, *My Sweet Dear*.

Favorite part of *Cielito Lindo* goes—

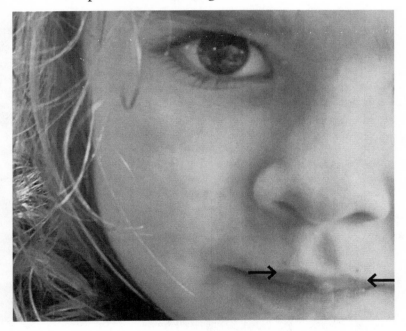

---

46 Yes, I know. Technically, two words. But "lovesong" can be one word, too. At least according to The Cure.

Ese lunar que tienes, cielito lindo
Junto a tu boca
No se lo des a nadie, cielito lindo
Que a mi me toca

A-ya-yayay, canta y no llores

Porque cantando se alegran, cielito lindo
Los corazones[47]

What took me so long. Am I too small a mother. Or my father too recently gone while as of yet undead. Too recently gone for me to share of father what is privately mine. In minuscule increments, I claw above.

For now, practice of paternal mariachi lovesong spreads. Little sweet dear mornings by my voice extend. For a moment, a parenthesis, an event of time, I feel I could not be more here with her, I who am her mother,   here.

Am I not.

( )

For a reason I can't quite fathom I get a circle tattoo. I see thin outline of empty, perfect circle on some stranger's calf & know I need one on my arm. On my own arm. A permanent mark bearing witness to empty space, that conduit between happened &   happening.

Often, I am asked—why the circle, what does it mean.

———

47 A laidback translation:

That mole you have, my sweet dear / by your mouth / give it to no one, my sweet dear / because it belongs to me. / A-ya-yayay, sing, don't cry / because by signing, my sweet dear / hearts fill with joy.

When I feel vague, I become voice who says—nothing in particular; it can mean anything.

When I feel generous, I become mouth who says—it can mean anything. I can just wake up and draw it in: planet, sun, soccer ball, apple, flower, happy, sad or startled face.

When I feel mystical, I become sound who says—what goes around comes around, I guess.

But, when I feel beaten, I do not become throat who says— round and round and round; over and over & over; again.

( )

Boy can handle the truth, says child psychologist who over several weeks spent hours with boy. *Give him the truth*, she says. *He doesn't fully understand what happened to him. What he sees is that all the doctors, all the treatments, didn't work. He thinks the doctors are stupid. From his eyes, what worked was the medication. How much have you told him.*

Well, he was with us obviously during all the different doctor consults, we say. *We always discussed everything in front of him. But you are right. We need to explain things better to him, probably use different terms. Do you think he has some form of trauma,* PTSD.

No. Not at all. He is just really, really confused. This confusion is generating quite a bit of anxiety. I think you can clear it up just by talking to him. Take your time. Have several sit downs. Honestly, I don't think you need me for this.

Okay. What about ADHD.

Listen, ADHD *describes a behavioral pattern. Sure, he has some of the elements of this pattern, some of the traits. Impulsivity, for example. But it's how you manage these traits that will determine his overall*

behavior. He responds very well to firm boundaries & incentives. I'll send
you a list of simple recommendations based on this.
 Okay. Thank you. Anything else we should do.
 Boy is great. He is fine. But he needs the truth.

( )

The truth of Guayaquil is this—
 There is no shortcut through the ten, the twenty, the many
years of parental toil. No ramp around. The only way is
through. Elsa who says our difficulties make us who we are.
Boy's overwrought brain is who he is. But who-ness of boy,
by transitive property of family, becomes who we are as parents as well. Who we are and who we endeavor, so hard, to be.
Via acceptance. Via unconditional love. Via application of
boundary, incentive, will. All the good stuff. All that fodder
of mature adult-life. All of it available here for us to—what's
the word—seize.
 Robert Frost who once, before all he wrote, quote by quote,
became remarkably oversold, said—

 ...the best way out is always through.
 And I agree to that, or in so far
 As that I can see no way out but through

(From 'A Servant to Servants')

The truth of everything else, or in so far as that I can see,
is this—

It happens. It happened. It's happening.

( )

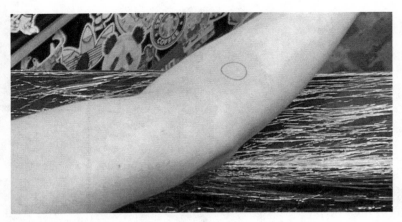

It happened on February 14, 1990—

An astronomer named Carl Sagan convinces NASA to turn the Voyageur I space probe around, just before probe exits boundaries of its communicable range, so that it can take one last shot of Earth as seen from the edge of solar system. One last flash with its last lamplight. In the photograph, Earth occupies less than one pixel, barely visible. Visible, only, according to Sagan, as a pale blue dot. Sagan writes a book about efforts required to obtain this image and what image represents, means, says, to him. In book, there is a section known as Sagan's "Pale Blue Dot Soliloquy."

I cannot go over, go beyond, mental image of years Sagan spends convincing NASA's super scientists to spin their super galactic probe around just before probe becomes eternally lost in space. Of probe spinning silently in space. Of probe finding, locating, exact right dot. Of Sagan, sitting still, in reverence, before the photo of his pale blue dot.

Of dot.

It is how I feel when I spin my head & see the book of words I've thrown into your open hands. *That's us.* That book.

That dot. All the nerves I threw in patterns on my screen. *That's here. That's home.*

Friend, mom of Anaya, shows me over coffee all the notepad entries on her phone. *I started writing down memories when Anaya got sick,* she says, *so I would be sure to keep them. Look at all the memories I have but only because I wrote them down.*

Keeping and having and holding and throwing. All a function of words we own, of names we name. Of will to say, to voice, to speak, to convey. Quote by quote, to tell—oh, to tell us all. Dot is so tiny. So tiny it cannot matter who first comes, who first names, but that we hop to it: to story: good, sad, so what. All becomes fact, becomes truth, once lettered words seize empty space of the page.

Give boy truth, therapist says. *He can handle truth. He is anxious, confused, because he does not have truth.*

What is truth if not the effort that produced this book.

Happy is for what. Rapture is for what. It is not event, not process, not happy, not sad, but book that is for what. Brown grey real-world transforms into remarkable healable matter via own words. Via book. It is book that we keep, have, hold. And that we hurl toward the next soul.

With words it happens: the unnamable is drawn, via shadow, called. I can say, *I sense it—that thing I do not, cannot, name.*

And.

With words it happens: I can say, *boy, my boy.*

Whose name is Lorenzo.

AUTHOR'S NOTES

Photographs

All the photos in this book, except for two, were taken by the me, the author Ana María Caballero. All photos are used in this book with the permission of any other person involved.

The photo of Jonathan Weinstein on p.33 was taken by Wendy Sewards who has kindly allowed me to include this picture of him.

The photos on p.138 of my son and his cousin were taken from the safety camera in my brother-in-law's house, and these are also used with permission.

Here is a list of the photos used in order:

Lorenzo with EEG Lying on Hospital Bed, Holter Monitor, Lithuania Phone Call Screen, Jonathan Weinstein, Lorenzo at Pedro Carmona's office, Statue of Virgin in the Office of the Veterinarian, Shelf in Veterinarian's Office, Nina in Aquarium, My Father's Hands, Lorenzo's Hands, My Hands, Lorenzo in Elsa Lucia's Home, Lorenzo with Elizabeth, Lorenzo's Seizure in Uncle's Kitchen. Lorenzo at Dr. Bravo's Office, Notes Drawn on Genetic Test, Pictures of Lorenzo's Medicines, Mayo Clinic Visit, Close up of Nina's Moles, My Tattoo.

Other Exhibits where permission has been granted

p.14 and p.26 Clips from my son's medical records. These are brief and are included for the sake of factual accuracy. My husband has agreed for these to be included.

p.91 Dr. Elsa Lucia Arango, for this doctor's note

p.255 Anaya's mother, for the text messages with myself

ACKNOWLEDGEMENTS

I am deeply grateful to everyone who appears by name in this manuscript. All of you, all of you, all of you, played a role in my son's recovery. But there are also many to whom I owe so much and who are not mentioned by name—first and foremost, Julie Marie Wade, my mentor.

Julie, for so many years I prayed out loud for a mentor, and the universe responded with you. Thank you, Julie. In your classroom I learned to believe in my voice and in my story. Without your guidance and enthusiasm, this book would not exist. I know I am not alone in feeling that your support transformed my path as a writer. I know I am not alone in thanking the universe for you.

I'm also forever grateful to all the doctors, medical practitioners and healers who committed their time and energy to finding a cure for our son's seizures. Elsa Lucia Arango, one of the busiest people I know, instantly responded to every single message, call, email we sent her with desperate questions. Sergio placed all his knowledge and contacts at our disposal. Lucy prayed daily for Lorenzo. Elizabeth, as she always did, devoted herself to thinking openly and thoroughly about what could be ailing our son. Elizabeth died of COVID, and this book is dedicated to her. I miss her so much. I sense her so much.

I also need to thank my in-laws, Jenaro and Rosi, with all my heart. They welcomed us in Bogotá for weeks during our son's treatments and took great care to prepare every one of his meals. What's more, they made sure he ate the green food on his plate.

To my husband Nelson David, I couldn't have gone through this experience with anyone else. The coffee we drank sustained us, sure, but more so our shared sense of humor, which, in my mind, beats the same name as love.

Last but certainly not least, I want to very specially thank everyone at The Black Spring Press Group, in particular Todd Swift, Amira Ghanim and Catherine Myddleton-Evans, for their incredible work in helping to bring my book into the world. I also want to thank Lisa Pasold, the judge of The 2020 International Beverly Prize for Literature, who selected my book for the press, changing my life forever.

WORKS CITED

Though not all these works are quoted in this text, each weighed heavily on my mind as I lived through my son's illness and wrote the pages of this book.

Cervantes Saavedra, Miguel de. 1547–1616. *The Adventures of Don Quixote de la Mancha*. New York: Farrar, Straux, Giroux, 1986.

Cohen, Leonard. 'Bird on a Wire.' *Songs from a Room,* 1969.

D'Agata, John. *The Next American Essay*. Graywolf Press, 2003.

Eliot, T.S., 'Preludes,' *Prufrock and Other Observations*, 1917.

Eliot, T.S., 'The Love Song of J. Alfred Prufrock,' *Prufrock and Other Observations*, 1917.

Hoang, Lily. *A Bestiary*. Cleveland State University Poetry Center, 2016.

Keats, John. Ode on Melancholy, 1820.

Lispector, Clarice. *La vida íntima de Laura*. V&R Ediciones, 2014.

Lispector, Clarice. *Near to the Wild Heart*. Translated by Giovanni Ponteiro. New Directions, 1990.

Rankine, Claudia, *Don't Let Me Be Lonely*. Penguin Books, 2017.

Reines, Ariana. *Mercury*. Fence Books, 2011.

Rulfo, Juan. *Aire de las colinas, Cartas a Clara*, Editorial Sud-americana, 2000.

Sacks, Oliver. *Gratitude*. Knopf, 2015.

Simic, Charles. *Sixty Poems*. Mariner Books, 2008.

Warhol, Andy. *The Philosophy of Andy Warhol (From A to B and Back Again)*. Harvest, 1977.